Meniere's Disease—
What You Need to Know

By P. J. Haybach, R.N., M.S.

Jerry L. Underwood, Ph.D., Editor

The Vestibular Disorders Association (VEDA) is a nonprofit organization that provides information and support to people with inner ear disorders. Founded in Portland, Oregon, in 1983, VEDA distributes information worldwide about the inner ear, the human balance system, Meniere's disease, benign paroxysmal positional vertigo (BPPV), labyrinthitis and related topics through its many publications, its site on the World Wide Web of the Internet, and its quarterly newsletter, On the Level. Contact VEDA for more information or to become a member.

Printed in the United States of America.

Published by the Vestibular Disorders Association
PO Box 4467
Portland, OR 97208-4467
(800) 837-8428
veda@vestibular.org
http://www.vestibular.org

First Edition
First Printing, August 1998; Second Printing, February 1999
Printed in the United States of America
10 9 8 7 6 5 4 3 2

International Standard Book Number: 0-9632611-1-8 (softcover)
0-9632611-2-6 (hardcover)

Table of Contents

Preface

We have written this book to fill the need for a basic work, understandable to the public, about Meniere's disease.

Our material is not limited to one viewpoint or approach to the disease. Instead, we have presented facts about Meniere's disease, pros and cons about various treatments, and a wide variety of viewpoints expressed by other authors, researchers, health professionals, and people who have been diagnosed with Meniere's disease.

We hope that our audience, after reading this book, will be well-informed about Meniere's disease, its symptoms and signs, vestibular testing, treatment options, coping strategies, and related issues. We also intend that our book be used to help educate family, friends, co-workers, employers, and others about the disease.

This book is not meant to substitute for professional health care or to promote or reject a particular theory or treatment.

Dedication

This book is dedicated to Judy Metroka, Michael La Porta and Rosemary Gellene for all they taught me about the pursuit of clinical excellence.

Acknowledgments

This book would not have been possible without the assistance of a great many people and organizations, including the medical and scientific advisors and the board of directors of the Vestibular Disorders Association.

People who read and commented on parts of the manuscript at various stages included F. Owen Black, M.D.; James O. Chinnis, Jr., Ph.D.; Joel A. Goebel, M.D.; Timothy C. Hain, M.D.; Vicente Honrubia, M.D.; Fay B. Horak, Ph.D., P.T.; Jeffrey Kramer, M.D.; Julie K. Purdy, Ph.D.; Neil T. Shepard, Ph.D.; Charlotte L. Shupert, Ph.D.; Joyce Sherman; Kathleen C. Stoner, Pharm. D.; June O. Underwood, Ph.D., and Susan Zalewa Tupper, R.N., M.S.

Others who provided insights on specific issues related to Meniere's disease included Marian Girardi, M.A.; Susan J. Herdman, Ph.D., P.T.; Alec N. Salt, Ph.D.; and Dennis P. O'Leary, Ph.D.

Saumil N. Merchant, M.D., and Sumiko M. Goldbaum, B.S., of the NIDCD National Temporal Bone, Hearing and Balance Pathology Resource Registry contributed Chapter 36.

The reference librarians of the Pinellas Park branch of the Pinellas County (Florida) Library were instrumental in obtaining many of the reference works needed to write this book.

Joyce Sherman, co-owner of River Graphics, Portland, Oregon, designed the book and coordinated indexing and printing.

Barbara Pinzka, Partners Marketing Communications, assisted with promotion.

The index was prepared by Monica Luce.

Chapter 1

Introduction

We have written this book chiefly for people who have or suspect they have Meniere's disease and who want to know more about its diagnosis and treatment as well as strategies for coping with its effects.

In this book, you will find information about virtually every aspect of the disease, from the basic anatomy and workings of the inner ear to things you should know about doctors, insurance companies, and support groups. We have also covered symptoms and symptom cycles, the physical changes caused by the disease, the tests, the treatments, and some of the controversies associated with Meniere's disease. Along the way, we discuss research, prevention, and how to find out more from libraries, associations, and the Internet.

Meniere's disease varies greatly in its onset, duration, intensity, periodicity, and in other ways from person to person. Not all of the information in this book will apply to your particular case, but we hope this book will move you toward wise health-care decisions and improve your life.

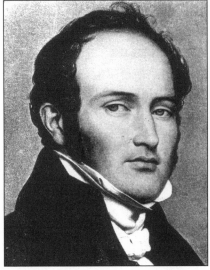

Prosper Meniere. (Courtesy of D. B. Pappas, M.D., Birmingham, Alabama)

History

Up until the late 1800s, people experiencing episodes of vertigo, tinnitus, and hearing loss were thought to have "apoplectiform cerebral congestion," an ill-defined brain problem. In 1861 Prosper Meniere, a French physician and director of the Imperial Institute for Deaf Mutes, presented a paper, "On a Particular Kind of Severe Hearing Loss Resulting from a Lesion of the Inner Ear," that for the first time linked these symptoms to the inner ear. Since that time, the name Meniere has been associated with this group of symptoms and sometimes, improperly, with inner ear problems in general.

What Is Meniere's Disease?

In this book, the term "Meniere's disease" will be used as defined in 1994 by the Committee on Hearing and Equilibrium of the American Academy of Otolaryngology-Head and Neck Surgery in the committee's guidelines for the diagnosis and evaluation of therapy for Meniere's disease.

Definition: The committee defines Meniere's disease as the "idiopathic syndrome of endolymphatic hydrops." This means that **Meniere's disease** has no known cause (is idiopathic), is characterized by a group of signs and symptoms, and is thought to be associated with endolymphatic hydrops, an abnormal enlargement of the innermost of the two fluid-filled spaces of the inner ear. Unfortunately this enlargement cannot be seen or measured with absolute certainty during the lifetime of a human being.

When the diagnosis of Meniere's disease is made, the presence of endolymphatic hydrops is suspected. Under the published guidelines, a case of Meniere's disease should not be reported in a scientific journal unless hearing loss and multiple attacks of spontaneous (unprovoked) vertigo, are present along with either tinnitus (noises in the ear) or aural fullness (fullness or pressure felt in the ear) all in the same ear.

Definition: Vertigo is the perception of movement (either of yourself or of objects around you) that is not occurring or is occurring differently from what you perceive.

Definition: Tinnitus, commonly referred to as ringing in the ears, means any abnormal noises in the ears.

In the past, many physicians included loss of consciousness as a symptom of Meniere's disease. The current definition of the disease, however, does not include loss of consciousness. Even so, it is commonly accepted that some people with Meniere's disease experience a feeling of faintness even if they do not faint.

Just as there is no known cause for Meniere's disease, there is no known cure or method, medical or surgical, to reverse the physical changes related to it within the inner ear. This does not mean the symptoms can't be treated, made better, or stopped. Many of its symptoms eventually stop spontaneously or with minimal treatment in the majority of people who have the disease. In addition, with the possible exception of falls or accidents caused by vertigo or the sudden and complete loss of balance sometimes associated with the disease, Meniere's disease is not fatal.

Controversy

Unfortunately, Meniere's disease is controversial in many ways. To begin with, even the correct spelling and use of accent marks with Meniere's name are not agreed upon. Meniere apparently wrote his name Menière, but his son used Ménière, which has become the accepted spelling. In this book, we usually use the Anglicized version, Meniere, without accents, which looks more familiar to U.S. readers but is not exactly correct.

Another controversy involves the choice of name for this condition and the meaning of the name. You will no doubt see or hear other terms being used that include the word "Meniere," such as Meniere's syndrome, triad of Meniere's, classic Meniere's, typical Meniere's, atypical Meniere's, cochlear Meniere's, vestibular Meniere's, Meniere's symptom complex, and Morbus Meniere. Their use is not formally regulated by any organization or agency. Confusion about their meaning often occurs. None of the other terms is defined by the committee, and we generally will not use them except to list them here.

A feature of the committee's definition is that since Meniere's disease is defined as idiopathic (of unknown cause), if the cause of your symptoms becomes known, by definition you no longer have Meniere's disease. This means that a diagnosis of Meniere's disease is somewhat tentative and perhaps temporary.

Many doctors speculate that Meniere's disease is not a single entity and may in fact be a name used for a number of different conditions. Future research and study may help resolve this issue and related questions about diagnostic methods and about treatments, particularly surgical treatments.

Numbers

Statistics about vestibular disorders and about Meniere's disease are hard to come by. However, *A Report of the Task Force on the National Strategic Research Plan* of the National Institute on Deafness and Other Communication Disorders (NIDCD), published in 1989, says that "over 90 millions Americans, age 17 and older, have experienced a dizziness or balance problem." The NIDCD is a part of the United States National Institutes of Health (NIH), and is based in Bethesda, Maryland. A more recent NIDCD report says that in the U.S. "approximately two million adults have chronic impairment from a dizziness or balance problem" and that "dizziness is the most common reason for seeking medical care in the over-75-year age group." Estimates of the annual costs for medical care for balance disorders exceeds $1 billion in the U.S. alone, according to the NIDCD. A significant fraction of these numbers result from Meniere's disease.

Definition: Vestibular refers to the balance parts of the inner ear and related structures.

The exact number of people with Meniere's disease is difficult to measure accurately because no official reporting system exists. Numbers used by researchers differ from one report to the next and from one country to the next. The National Institutes of Health estimates that about 545,000 people in the U.S. have Meniere's disease and that 38,250 are diagnosed each year.

A Japanese study looking at one geographic area in Japan over a number of years estimated that 17 of every 100,000 people in the population would be diagnosed with Meniere's disease each year. An American study looked at Rochester, Minnestoa, from 1951 to 1980, and concluded that of every 100,000 people in the population 218.2 had Meniere's disease and 15.3 would be diagnosed with it each year.

Studies from Germany, Japan, and the U.S. show the most common age of a person starting out with Meniere's disease is 40-49. Slightly more women develop it than men.

According to various studies, between 60 percent and 80 percent of the people diagnosed with Meniere's disease will either get better on their own or will respond well to medical treatment. This majority will not need to apply for permanent disability or require surgical intervention.

The number of people who have Meniere's disease in one ear and who will ultimately develop the problem in both ears is also not known. Estimates range from 17.7 percent to 75 percent. The Rochester, Minnesota, study reported a 34 percent rate of bilateral disease over time.

Famous People and Meniere's

The list of well-known public figures who are thought to have had Meniere's disease includes Vincent Van Gogh, Martin Luther, Julius Caesar, Jonathan Swift, and Mamie Eisenhower (wife of U.S. President Dwight Eisenhower).

Of course, since the diagnosis of Meniere's disease didn't exist before the middle of the 19th century and since no one can examine, test, or talk to historical figures, a retrospective Meniere's diagnosis is open to debate.

In 1979, a Japanese doctor, K. Yasuda, asked in a medical journal, "Was Van Gogh suffering from Meniere's disease?" This article was followed in 1990 by another, "Van Gogh Has Meniere's Disease and Not Epilepsy," by multiple authors, and it was based on interpretations of many Van Gogh letters that seem to describe attacks of vertigo, nausea, vomiting, noise intolerance, tinnitus, fluctuating hearing loss, motion intolerance, and positional vertigo, with symptom-free periods. The speculation about Van Gogh and Meniere's disease was made even more interesting by the fact that Van Gogh cut off one of his ears.

Jonathan Swift, author of *Gulliver's Travels* and other literary works, first became ill with what was apparently Meniere's disease when he was in his 20s. He wrote about the symptoms and related problems in many letters. Despite the nearly life-long presence of Meniere's, he completed a doctorate in divinity, wrote books, carried out his duties as the Dean of St. Patrick's Cathedral in Dublin, and carried on a large volume of correspondence with a large number of people.

Terence Cawthorne, a British physician, suggested in 1957 that Julius Caesar might have had Meniere's disease rather than epilepsy, which others suspected Caesar might have had. Cawthorne's observation is based on only a few contemporary descriptions of Julius Caesar as having had the "falling sickness" and a line written by Shakespeare referring to Caesar's apparent loss of hearing in one ear.

Using Reference Sections

Most of the chapters in this book include a reference list of books and articles used in preparation of the chapter and/or that you might find interesting. In the case of "Part III: Examination and Testing," a combined reference list appears at the end of Chapter 18, "Future Tests."

For journal citations, the names are those of the author or authors, if known; the article name appears in quotes; the title of the journal is italicized; the first number is the volume number (usually representing the number of years the journal has been published); the number, if any, in parentheses is the issue number (many times representing the number of the month); the next numbers are the page numbers in the journal where you can find the article, and the last number is the year of publication.

For books, the names are those of the author or authors (if known); the book title appears in italics; then comes the city of publication, the publishing company's name, and the date of publication.

Disclaimer

The information in this book is not intended as a substitute for professional health care. Before acting on any information found in this book, you should discuss it with your personal physician.

Neither VEDA nor the author advocate any particular course of treatment for any particular disorder.

References

_____. *A Report of the Task Force on the National Strategic Research Plan (1989)*. Bethesda, Md.: National Institute on Deafness and Other Communication Disorders.

_____. "Committee on Hearing and Equilibrium Guidelines for the Diagnosis and Evaluation of Therapy in Meniere's Disease." *Otolaryngology—Head and Neck Surgery*, 113(3): 181-185, 1995.

_____. *National Strategic Research Plan for Balance and the Vestibular System and Language and Language Impairments (1991)* (NIH Publication No. 91-3217). Bethesda, Md.: National Institute on Deafness and Other Communication Disorders.

_____. *National Strategic Research Plan 1991, 1992, 1993* (NIH Publication No. 95-3711). Bethesda, Md.: National Institute on Deafness and Other Communication Disorders.

_____. *National Strategic Research Plan 1994-1995: Language and Language Impairments, Balance and Balance Disorders, Voice and Voice Disorders (*NIH Publication No. 96-3217*)*. Bethesda, Md.: National Institute on Deafness and Other Communication Disorders (NIDCD).

Arenberg, I.K. "A Clinical Analysis of Prosper Meniere's Original Cases." *American Journal of Otology*, 10(4):314-326, 1989.

Arenberg, I.K., Countryman, L.F., Bernstein, L.H., and Shambaugh, G.E. "Van Gogh Had Meniere's Disease and Not Epilepsy." *Journal of the American Medical Association*, 264(4): 491-493, 1990.

Atkinson, M. "Meniere's Original Papers." *Acta Otolaryngologica, Supplement*, 162, 1961.

Beasley, N.J., and Jones, N.S. "Meniere's Disease: Evaluation of a Definition." *Journal of Laryngology and Otology*, 110:1107-1113, 1996.

Brookes, G.B. "Meniere's Disease: A Practical Approach to Management." *Drugs*, 25:77-89, 1983.

Brown, J.S. "A Ten Year Statistical Follow-Up of 245 Consecutive Cases of Endolymphatic Shunt and Decompression with 328 Consecutive Cases of Labyrinthectomy." *Laryngoscope*, 93:1419-1424, 1983.

Cawthorne, T.E. "Julius Caesar and the Falling Sickness." *Proceedings of the Royal Society of Medicine*, 51:27-30, 1957.

Chalat, N.I. "Who Was Prosper Meniere and Why Am I Still So Dizzy?" *American Journal of Otology*, 1(1):52-56, 1979.

Pappas, D.G., and McGuinn, M.G. "Unpublished Letters from Prosper Meniere: A Personal Silhouette." *American Journal of Otology*, 14(4):318-325, 1993.

Schuknecht, H.F. *Pathology of the Ear*. Cambridge, Mass.: Harvard University Press, 1974.

Shapiro, S.L. "The Medical History of Jonathan Swift." *The Ear, Nose, and Throat Monthly*, 48:97-100, 1969.

Watanabe, Y., Mizukoshi, K., Shojaku, H., Watanabe, I., Hinoki, M., and Kitahara, M. "Epidemiological and Clinical Characteristics of Meniere's Disease in Japan." *Acta Otolaryngologica, Supplement*, 519, 206-210, 1995.

Wladislavosky-Waserman, P., Facer, G.W., Mokri, B., and Kurland, L.T. "Meniere's Disease: a 30-Year Epidemiologic and Clinical Study in Rochester, Minn., 1951-1980." *Laryngoscope*, 94, 1098-1102, 1984.

Yasuda, K. "Was Van Gogh Suffering from Meniere's Disease?" *Otalgia*, 25:1427-1439, 1979.

Part I:
Anatomy
and
Physiology

To understand the ear, what goes wrong with it, where various symptoms come from, and how different treatments work in Meniere's disease, you should understand something about the ear's normal structure (anatomy) and function (physiology).

Chapter 2

The Normal Ear

T he ear is involved in two important but quite different functions, hearing and balance, and it is divided into three general
parts, the external ear, the middle ear, and the inner ear. These
are shown in Figure 2-1.

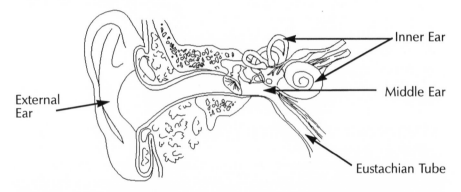

Figure 2-1: The ear. Note the three general parts: the external ear, the middle ear, and the inner ear. (From LifeArt, Corel Gallery Collection, Copyright
© 1994, Williams and Wilkins, a Waverly company, with permission.)

External Ear

The external ear has three regions—the outside flap (called the
auricle or pinna), the ear canal or external auditory canal, and the
canal side of the ear drum (also called the tympanic membrane).

The external ear is involved in hearing but not balance. Sound, in
the form of sound (air pressure) waves, is collected and slightly ampli-
fied by the auricle and funneled into the ear via the external auditory
canal. The vibration of the sound waves causes the tympanic membrane
to move in and out, and the sound waves are passed to the middle ear.

Middle Ear

The middle ear cavity is basically an air-filled space. It contains the other side of the ear drum, three small bones, and the opening of the eustachian tube.

The main function of the middle ear is to transmit sound vibrations from the air-filled external ear via solid bones and membranes to the fluid-filled inner ear.

The middle ear contains three little bones called the ossicles. These include the malleus, incus, and stapes, also known as the hammer, anvil, and stirrup. The flat area of the innermost bone, the stapes, is called the stapes footplate, and it rests in the oval window, a membrane-covered opening into the inner ear.

Generally speaking, a diagnosis of "fluid in the ears" means that an abnormal collection of fluid is present in the middle ear cavity.

The eustachian tube is an hourglass-shaped tube connecting the middle ear with the area of the throat behind the nose. Its function is to allow air pressure to be equal on both sides of the tympanic membrane. This is important because if the pressure on one side of the membrane is higher than the other, pain and damage can occur. The eustachian tube is usually closed but opens during swallowing and yawning, allowing pressure equalization to occur.

The mastoid is a bone, partly filled with air spaces, located behind the ear.

Two openings, the oval window and the round window, connect the middle ear and the inner ear. The round window is covered with a membrane. The oval window is covered by a membrane and the footplate of the stapes and is surrounded by an annular (ring-shaped) ligament.

Inner Ear

The inner ear, unlike the other regions of the ear, is involved in both hearing and balance and is the part of the ear affected by

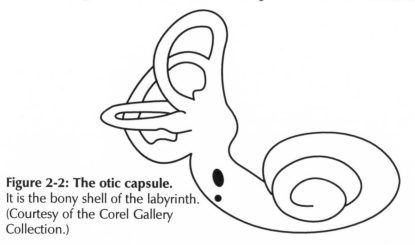

Figure 2-2: The otic capsule.
It is the bony shell of the labyrinth.
(Courtesy of the Corel Gallery
Collection.)

Meniere's disease. It is fluid-filled and encased in the temporal bone (the densest bone in the body and one of the bones of the skull). The inner ear includes two compartments, one inside the other (the bony labyrinth and the membranous labyrinth), three connected sensory regions (the semicircular canals, vestibule, and cochlea), and the endolymphatic sac and duct.

The outer shell of the bony labyrinth, called the otic capsule, can be seen in Figure 2-2. (If the inner ear could be removed intact from its place within the temporal bone, it would appear like this.)

The bony labyrinth consists of the otic capsule and the space between the otic capsule and the membranous labyrinth. This space is filled with perilymph, one of the two inner ear fluids. The perilymph surrounds, cushions, and is considered part of the membranous labyrinth, shown in Figure 2-3.

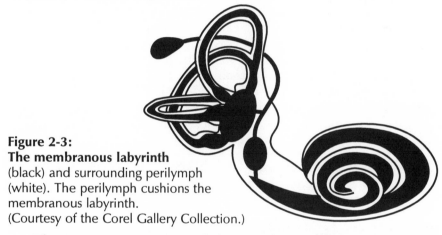

Figure 2-3:
The membranous labyrinth
(black) and surrounding perilymph
(white). The perilymph cushions the
membranous labyrinth.
(Courtesy of the Corel Gallery Collection.)

The inner compartment of the membranous labyrinth is filled with endolymph, the other of the two inner ear fluids. The membranous labyrinth also contains the hair cells, which detect sound waves, movement, and gravity. In Meniere's disease an abnormally large amount of endolymph is thought to be present within the membranous labyrinth.

Note: Although both inner ear fluids end in "lymph," they are not part of the lymphatic system. The prefix "endo" stands for "within," and the prefix "peri" stands for "around."

The inner ear is sometimes referred to as the "labyrinth" because of the maze of tiny passageways and winding structures, which become apparent when you look at a diagram of the membranous labyrinth. See Figure 2-3.

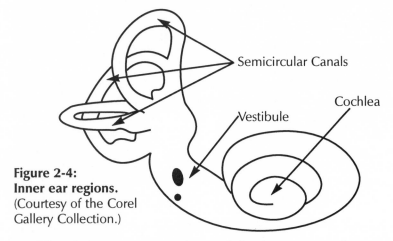

Figure 2-4:
Inner ear regions.
(Courtesy of the Corel
Gallery Collection.)

The three sensory regions of the inner ear—the semicircular canals, vestibule, and cochlea—are shown in Figure 2-4.

The function of the inner ear is to convert mechanical energy (sound waves, movement, and gravity information) acting on inner ear hair cells into nerve signals. All of the hair cells within the semicircular canals, vestibule, and cochlea are found inside the membranous labyrinth. Hearing hair cells are found inside in the cochlea, and balance hair cells are found inside in the semicircular canals and the vestibule. Each hair cell has 60 to 80 submicroscopic "hairs" called cilia protruding from its surface.

Definition: A **hair cell** is a cylindrical cell which has cilia (hairlike projections) protruding from one end.

Semicircular Canals

You have six semicircular canals, three in each ear. The canals are embedded in the temporal bone of the skull and move when your head moves. The three canals in each ear lie perpendicular to one another, each in a different plane. (The end wall, side wall, and floor of a typical room in a house are perpendicular to one another, each in a different plane.) Figure 2-5 will give you an idea of how the canals lie in relation to one another.

The semicircular canals have technical names in medical texts. The anterior canal is also referred to as the superior canal. The lateral canal is also referred to as the horizontal canal, and the posterior canal may also be referred to as the inferior vertical canal. In an upright human, the anterior and posterior canals are vertical in relation to the head, and the horizontal is horizontal.

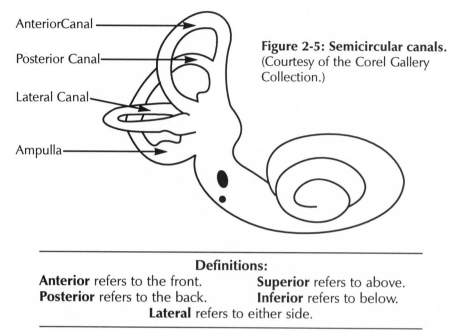

AnteriorCanal

Posterior Canal

Lateral Canal

Ampulla

Figure 2-5: Semicircular canals.
(Courtesy of the Corel Gallery Collection.)

Definitions:

Anterior refers to the front.   **Superior** refers to above.
Posterior refers to the back.   **Inferior** refers to below.
Lateral refers to either side.

At the end of each semicircular canal is a widened area called the ampulla (plural ampullae). See Figure 2-5.

Each ampulla houses the cupula and balance hair cells of its semicircular canal. The three paddle-shaped ampullae of each ear collectively contain approximately 23,000 hair cells. These hair cells are gathered in a group within the membranous labyrinth and are covered by a gelatinous-like substance. This group of cells is referred to as the crista or crista ampullaris, and the gelatinous mass is called the cupula.

Because of their structure, the semicircular canals are responsible for sensing rotational head movement (or rotational body movement that includes the head). When you turn your head, the endolymph fluid lags in the affected canal, creating pressure against its cupula. The resulting distortion of the cupula moves the hair cells, which secrete a neurotransmitter (chemical) that causes a nerve signal to be sent to the brain.

Vestibule

The vestibule is the region of the inner ear between the cochlea and the semicircular canals. It contains two balance organs, the saccule and the utricle. Together they are referred to as the otolithic organs. They can be seen in Figure 2-6.

Each otolithic organ contains hair cells gathered together in an area called the macula (plural maculae). The tops of these hair cell groups are covered with and attached to a gelatinous substance with

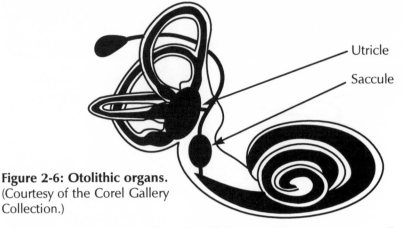

Utricle

Saccule

Figure 2-6: Otolithic organs.
(Courtesy of the Corel Gallery
Collection.)

calcium carbonate crystals embedded in it. This covering is called the otolithic membrane. The calcium carbonate crystals are called "otoliths" and sometimes "ear rocks." The macula of the saccule and the macula of the utricle lie at right angles to one another. Each ear contains a total of about 4,000 balance hair cells in the otolithic organs. Because they are weighted on top by the otoliths, the thousands of hair cells in these organs are affected by head movement in a straight line and by gravity.

Although each vestibule contains only two of the five balance end organs found in each ear, the word "vestibular" refers to all five.

Cochlea

The cochlea is the end organ of hearing. It is similar to a length of tubing or hose that has been coiled 2¾ times from the wide "bottom" or base to the narrow "top" or apex. The shape is like a snail's shell, hence the name "cochlea," which is Latin for snail.

One row of inner hair cells and three rows of outer hair cells run the entire length of the cochlea. Each ear has approximately 16,000 hair cells that cannot be replaced if lost.

When a turn of the cochlea is sliced crosswise to allow viewing of the inside, you can see three large fluid-filled tubes separated by two membranes. See Figure 2-7.

The three fluid-filled tubes are the scala vestibuli, the scala tympani, and, between them, the scala media, also called the cochlear duct. Both the scala tympani and the scala vestibuli are filled with perilymph, and the scala media is filled with endolymph. The upper membrane is Reissner's membrane, and the lower is the basilar membrane.

Definition: A **membrane** is a thin layer of tissue that separates one body compartment from another. Reissner's membrane separates the scala vestibuli from the scala media.

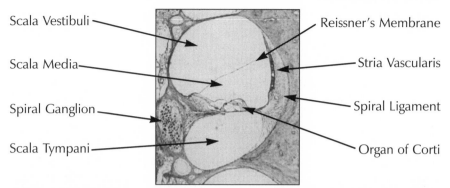

Scala Vestibuli

Scala Media

Spiral Ganglion

Scala Tympani

Reissner's Membrane

Stria Vascularis

Spiral Ligament

Organ of Corti

Figure 2-7: Cochlear cross-section. (Courtesy of Alec N. Salt, Ph.D., Washington University School of Medicine, St. Louis, Missouri, with permission.)

In addition to being the end organ of hearing, the cochlea also manufactures the inner ear fluid called endolymph. This is done in the stria vascularis, shown in Figure 2-7. (In addition, cells known as "dark cells" in the balance organs are thought to make endolymph.)

Endolymphatic Sac and Duct

The endolymphatic duct and sac can be seen leading away from the inner ear toward the covering of the brain in Figure 2-8.

The endolymphatic duct and sac are part of the membranous labyrinth in a space outside the bony labyrinth. Traditionally the endolymphatic sac has been thought to reabsorb the endolymph produced by the inner ear after it has flowed through the ear. If the excess endolymph thought to be associated with Meniere's disease were caused by a reabsorption defect, the problem would be right here.

The normal sac actually lies between the temporal bone and the

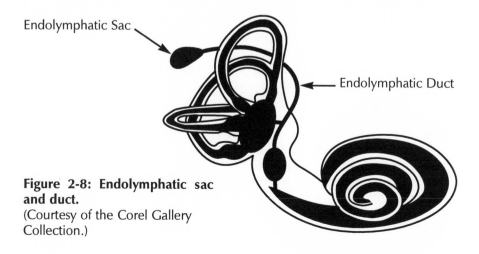

Endolymphatic Sac

Endolymphatic Duct

Figure 2-8: Endolymphatic sac and duct.
(Courtesy of the Corel Gallery Collection.)

brain rather than totally inside the temporal bone like the other parts of the inner ear. A portion of the sac is wrapped in the dura mater, the outermost layer of the brain's protective covering, the meninges. One type of surgery for Meniere's disease involves inserting a device in the sac or duct in an attempt to allow the endolymph to drain away.

In some people with Meniere's disease, the endolymphatic sac can be of quite different shapes and sizes with locations varying from one person to the next. In some of these people, the sacs are located entirely within the temporal bone, and in others they actually extend slightly beyond temporal bone into the cavity holding the brain. (This variability makes finding this structure during surgery difficult at times.)

The endolymphatic sac has been found by some researchers and surgeons to be smaller than average in people with Meniere's disease.

Note: Calling this structure a sac makes the structure seem simpler than it is. It is not shaped like a balloon; it is more like a series of passageways or caves.

The functions of the sac are not totally known or understood but probably include endolymph reabsorption, secretion of chemicals to assist in movement of endolymph through the inner ear, immune functions (as a defense organ to protect the ear from disease), ridding the endolymph of waste products, and possibly endolymph production.

Definition: To **secrete** is to pass a substance, not a waste product, produced within the cell to outside that cell. (To **excrete** would be to eliminate waste products.)

Other Structures

In addition to the three sensory regions (semicircular canals, vestibule, and cochlea) and the two containers of the inner ear (the bony labyrinth and membranous labyrinth), a handful of other important structures are associated with the inner ear including the vestibulo-cochlear nerve, the internal auditory canal, and the vestibular dark cells.

Balance and hearing information collected by the inner ear can't be used unless it reaches the brain. This information travels to the brain along the eighth cranial nerve, also called the vestibulo-cochlear nerve, cochleo-vestibular nerve, auditory nerve, or acoustic nerve. In this book, we use the term "vestibulo-cochlear nerve," which states the dual purpose of the nerve. Two branches of this nerve leave the inner ear, the vestibular branch and the cochlear branch; the vestibular branch carries vestibular messages from the five balance end organs, and the cochlear branch carries cochlear messages from the organ of Corti.

Definition: A **cranial nerve** is a nerve that originates in the brain and travels to a specific body area without running through the spinal cord. There are 12 pairs of cranial nerves carrying information to the brain and from the brain to help accomplish an astonishing number of functions including vision, balance, and hearing.

The vestibulo-cochlear nerve travels from the ear to the brain inside a tunnel called the internal auditory canal (IAC). Another nerve, the facial nerve, also travels to the brain through this canal.

Dark cells can be found in many areas of the vestibular membranous labyrinth. The function of these areas is thought to be endolymph production and fluid movement within the inner ear.

References

_____. American Academy of Otolaryngology—Head and Neck Surgery. "Earache and Otitis Media" (brochure), 1995.

Ammirati, M., Spallone, A., Feghali, J., Cheatham, M., and Becker, D. "The Endolymphatic Sac: Microsurgical Topographic Anatomy." *Neurosurgery*, 36(2), 416-419, 1995.

Anson, B.J. and Donaldson, J.A. *Surgical Anatomy of the Temporal Bone*. Philadelphia: W.B. Saunders Company, 1981.

Bagger-Sjoback, D. "Surgical Anatomy of the Endolymphatic Sac." *American Journal of Otology*, 14(6), 576-579, 1993.

Baloh, R.W. and Honrubia, V. *Clinical Neurophysiology of the Vestibular System*. Philadelphia: F.A. Davis Company, 1979.

Berne, R.M., and Levy, M.N. *Physiology*. Third edition. St Louis: Mosby YearBook, 1993.

Cummings, C.W., and Harker, L.A. *Otolaryngology—Head and Neck Surgery*. St. Louis: Mosby, 1992.

Dereberry, M.J. "Allergic and Immunologic Aspects of Meniere's Disease." *Otolaryngology—Head and Neck Surgery*, 114, 360-365, 1996.

Guyton, A.C. and Hall, J.E. *Textbook of Medical Physiology*. Philadelphia: W.B. Saunders Company, 1996.

Hebbar, G.K., Rask-Andersen, G., and Linthicum, F.H. "Three-Dimensional Analysis of 61 Human Endolymphatic Ducts and Sacs in Ears with and without Meniere's Disease." *Annals of Otology, Rhinology, and Laryngology*, 100, 219-225, 1991.

Jacobson, G.P., Newman, C.W. and Kartush, J.M. *Handbook of Balance Function Testing*. St. Louis: Mosby Year Book, 1993.

Jansson, B. and Rask-Andersen, H. "Erythrocyte Removal and Blood Clearance in the Endolymphatic Sac." *Acta Otolaryngologica*, 116, 429-434, 1996.

Ludman, H. *Mawson's Diseases of the Ear.* Fifth edition. Chicago: Year Book Medical Publishers, Inc., 1988.

Marieb, E.N. *Human Anatomy and Physiology*. Third edition. Redwood City, Calif.: The Benjamin/Cummings Publishing Company Inc., 1995.

Northern, J.L. *Hearing Disorders*. Second edition. Boston: Allyn and Bacon, 1984.

Proctor, B. *Surgical Anatomy of the Ear and Temporal Bone*. New York: Thieme Medical Publishers, Inc., 1989.

Snell, R.S. *Clinical Anatomy for Medical Students*. Fifth edition. Boston: Little, Brown and Company, 1995.

Schmidt, F.R. and Thews, G. *Human Physiology*. New York: Springer-Verlag, 1989.

Soliman, A.M. "A Subpopulation of Meniere's Patients Produce Antibodies That Bind to Endoymphatic Sac Antigens." *American Journal of Otology*, 17, 76-80, 1996.

Thibodeau, G.A., and Patton, K.T. "Sense Organs." *Anatomy and Physiology*. Second edition. St. Louis: Mosby Book Company, 1993.

Thomas, C.L. *Taber's Cyclopedic Medical Dictionary*. Fifteenth edition. Philadelphia: F.A. Davis Company, 1985.

Tortora, G.J., and Grabowski, S.R. *Principles of Anatomy and Physiology*. Seventh edition. New York: HarperCollins College Publishers, 1993.

University of Texas Medical Branch, Grand Rounds, Dept. of Otolaryngology. "Vestibular Anatomy and Physiology." http://www.ears.com. Oct. 4, 1996.

University of Wisconsin, Neurophysiology. "General Structure and Development of the External Ear, Middle Ear and Inner Ear; Hearing and Balance; Objective 6: Blood Supply to the Inner Ear." http://www.neurophys.wisc.edu?h&b/textbook/general_structure.html." Nov. 15, 1996.

Welling, D.B., Pasha, R., Roth, L.J., and Barin, K. "The Effect of Endolymphatic Sac Excision in Meniere's Disease." *American Journal of Otology*, 17, 278-282, 1996.

Chapter 3

Hearing

Unlike vestibular disorders such as BPPV, which affects only the balance-related structures of the inner ear, Meniere's disease affects hearing as well as balance.

Before you can hear anything, there must be sound. Sound begins as vibration. Striking a drum, blowing into a clarinet, shutting a door, ringing a bell, and speaking all create vibrations. These vibrations are transferred into their surroundings—air, liquid, or solid—where they take the form of sound or, more properly, sound waves.

In depth (sound waves): Movement of molecules is begun by vibration and becomes sound waves. These molecules bunch up in one area, and this causes the molecules in adjacent areas to be further apart. Each vibration creates a separate sound wave; there are as many sound waves as there are vibrations.

Definition: A **molecule** is the smallest amount of a substance that can keep the characteristics of the substance. One molecule of H_2O (two atoms of hydrogen attached to one atom of oxygen) is the smallest possible amount of water. Broken down further, the molecule becomes separate hydrogen atoms and an oxygen atom, not water.

Hearing

Sound waves can enter your inner ear and be heard either by air conduction or bone conduction.

During air conduction, the sound wave, helped somewhat by the pinna of your outer ear, enters your external auditory canal and strikes your tympanic membrane (ear drum). The membrane begins to vibrate, moving in and out (toward your middle ear and then toward your external auditory canal). Your ear drum vibrates at the same frequency as the sound wave. The greater the amplitude or intensity, the further your tympanic membrane actually moves.

Because the malleus is attached to the tympanic membrane, it also vibrates. This vibration spreads to the incus and then to the stapes. The end of the stapes, the stapes footplate, pushes in and pulls out of the oval window, a membrane-covered opening into your inner ear.

Bone conduction occurs with louder sounds when sound waves cause the bones of your skull to vibrate. This vibration does two things; it causes the fluid and structures of the cochlea to vibrate, and it also causes vibration of the ossicular chain and transmission of the vibration into the cochlea via the oval window.

Bone conduction is not very important in your everyday life; you rely upon air conduction much more. The sounds you hear by bone conduction have a somewhat different quality then those traveling through air. For example, a tape recording of your voice sounds much different to you than the sound you hear when you hear yourself speaking (via bone conduction).

Whatever route sound waves take, they must become a movement in the cochlear fluid before you can hear them. As described in the previous chapter, the cochlea has three channels running from its base (the wide part closest to the middle ear) to its apex. The three channels are the scala vestibuli, scala tympani, and scala media (also called the cochlear duct). The sound wave enters the scala vestibuli via the oval window and causes a wave of movement along the basilar membrane from base to apex. This moving wave is referred to as the traveling wave.

Note: *Scala* is Italian for staircase.

The pie-shaped area in the middle of Figure 3-1 is the scala media or cochlear duct. The scala media is part of the membranous labyrinth and has three "walls"—the stria vascularis, basilar membrane, and Reissner's membrane. Part of the scala media is the organ of Corti, which includes hair cells that detect the traveling wave.

Within the organ of Corti, the structure that is perhaps most important for hearing is the hair cell. The function of a cochlear hair

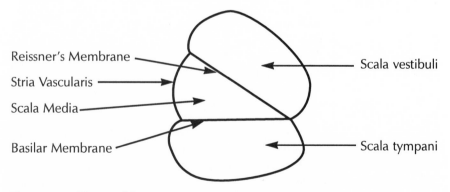

Figure 3-1: The cochlea.

cell is to convert mechanical energy from the traveling wave into an electrical signal. About 18,500 hair cells are arranged along the length of the cochlea. The cilia of the hair cells detect pressure changes as the traveling wave makes its way through the cochlea. The cells release a neurotransmitter, and electrical impulses or messages start on their way to your brain.

SOUND PATHWAY TO THE BRAIN

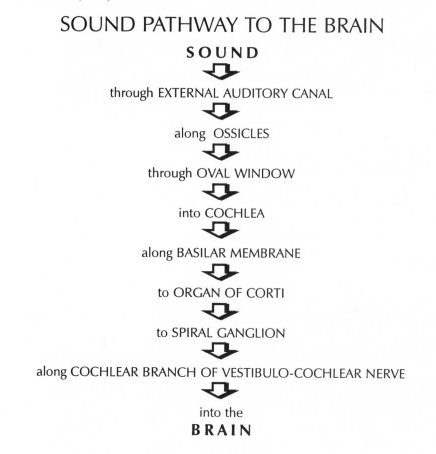

S O U N D

through EXTERNAL AUDITORY CANAL

along OSSICLES

through OVAL WINDOW

into COCHLEA

along BASILAR MEMBRANE

to ORGAN OF CORTI

to SPIRAL GANGLION

along COCHLEAR BRANCH OF VESTIBULO-COCHLEAR NERVE

into the
B R A I N

Cochlear Changes in Meniere's Disease

The two illustrations in Chapter 36, "Temporal Bone Bank," show a cross-section of a normal cochlea and a cross-section of the cochlear change thought to occur in the membranous labyrinth from an excessive amount of endolymph, a condition known as endolymphatic hydrops. (See Figure 36-1 and Figure 36-2, page 269.)

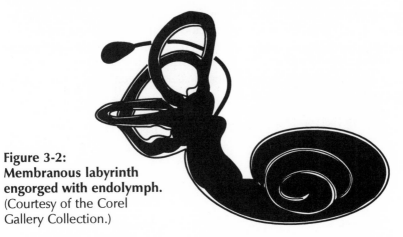

Figure 3-2:
Membranous labyrinth
engorged with endolymph.
(Courtesy of the Corel
Gallery Collection.)

Figure 3-2 shows how engorged with endolymph the membranous labyrinth can become.

History: In 1938, both a Japanese physician and two British physicians published the first papers describing endolymphatic hydrops in patients with Meniere's disease. The ear change was found by studying parts of the temporal bones with a microscope, something that could not be done during life. (Ears continue to be studied in this fashion. See Chapter 36 for more information about temporal bone research and donation.)

In severe cases, the cochlear duct enlargement can rupture Reissner's membrane and cause the potassium-rich endolymph and sodium-rich perilymph to mix. This release of potassium kills hair cells. It is not known if abnormal mixing of the two quite chemically different fluids causes the acute symptoms, including the attacks or hearing problems of Meniere's disease, but this is one of the theories.

One problem area: Not everyone with the diagnosis of Meniere's disease demonstrates ruptures, and some people with ruptures apparently do not have symptoms during their lifetime. Fifteen percent of presumptively normal individuals who have had their temporal bones studied have had hydrops in the apex area of the cochlea.

Some of the other possible changes seen with endolymphatic hydrops include compression and degeneration of the organ of Corti, degeneration of the stria vascularis, damage to the hair cells and their cilia, and a disturbance in the motion of the basilar membrane.

Information about hearing tests can be found in Chapter 15, "Hearing Tests."

References

Bern, R.M., and Levy, M.N. *Physiology.* Third edition. St. Louis: Mosby Yearbook. 1993.

Hallpike, C.S., and Cairns, H. "Observations on the Pathology of Meniere's Syndrome," *Journal of Laryngology and Otology,* 53:625-55. 1938.

Marieb, E.N. *Human Anatomy and Physiology.* New York: The Benjamin/Cummings Publishing Co. 1995.

Northern, J.L. *Hearing Disorders.* Second edition. Boston: Allyn and Bacon. 1984.

Rahn, J.E. *Ears, Hearing, and Balance.* New York: Atheneum. 1984.

Rauch, S.D., Merchant, S.N., and Thedinger, B.A. "Meniere's Syndrome and Endolymphatic Hydrops: Double Blind Temporal Bone Study," *Annals of Otology, Rhinology, and Laryngology,* 98:873-882. 1989.

Schmidt, R.F., and Thews, G. *Human Physiology.* New York: Springer-Verlag. 1989.

Thibodeau, G.A., and Patton, K.T. *Anatomy and Physiology.* Second edition. St. Louis: Mosby Book Co. 1993.

Thomas, C.L. *Taber's Cyclopedic Medical Dictionary.* Fifteenth Edition. Philadelphia: F.A. Davis Co. 1985.

Tortora, G.J., and Grabowski, S.R. *Principles of Anatomy and Physiology.* New York: Harper Collins College Publishers. 1993.

Balance and Other Vestibular Functions

Hearing is one sensory function of your inner ear. Providing vestibular information for balance, clear vision, a steady head, and some automatic body functions is the other.

Although less widely discussed and less understood than hearing, vestibular function is no less important. In fact, it may be easier to live with damaged hearing than with damaged vestibular function and therefore with a damaged sense of balance. So important is balance to normal functioning that it might best be regarded as the *sixth sense*, on a par with the five famous ones, sight, hearing, touch, taste, and smell.

Vestibular function includes the collection, transmission, and reflex use of movement, gravity, and position information. The vestibular apparatus of the inner ear, vestibulo-cochlear nerve, brain, and the vestibular reflexes are all involved.

Movement, Gravity, Position

The maculae of the saccule and utricle and the cristae of the semicircular canals are responsible for sensing position, head movement, and the effect of gravity. The job of these parts of your inner ear is to change the information they sense into biological signals or nerve impulses that can be sent to your brain and used for balance control.

The saccule and utricle (otolithic organs) are located in the vestibule, and one crista ampullaris (containing hair cells) is located in each of the three semicircular canals. The function of these parts is described below one at a time for clarity, but the "real-life" situation is far more complex than these examples. In reality, head movements affect multiple parts of both ears simultaneously.

Otolithic Organs

Each ear has a pair of organs, the saccule and utricle (otolithic organs), to sense both gravity and other linear accelerations of the head. The hair cells of the macula in each organ do this sensing.

Definition: Linear acceleration refers to a change in velocity along a straight line. An example of the sense of linear acceleration is the effect you feel when a jet airplane in which you are riding increases its speed as it zooms down the runway preparing for take-off.

Because they are weighted on top by the otoliths (calcium carbonate crystals), the thousands of hair cells in these organs are affected by head movement in a straight line and by gravity. When the otolithic membrane shifts position because of linear accelerations, the cilia are bent (sheared). This shearing causes an increase in information being sent to the brain. The hair cells of the otolithic organs send about 50-100 nerve pulses per second, a quantity the brain expects all the time. The brain uses other sensory information (e.g. visual) to correctly interpret the information from the otolithic organs.

Semicircular Canals

Because of their structure, the semicircular canals are responsible for sensing rotational head movement (or rotational body movement that includes the head). The canals move with head turns (angular acceleration), but the endolymphatic fluid in the affected canal lags, creating pressure against the cupula. The resulting distortion of the cupula moves the hair cells, which secrete a neurotransmitter (chemical) that causes a nerve signal to be sent to the brain. Gravity does not affect the canals if they are normal.

Definition: Angular acceleration refers to a change in velocity along a curved path such as a circle. An example of the sense of angular acceleration is the main vestibular effect you feel on a merry-go-round or spinning around on your feet while dancing or skating.

Like the otolithic organs, the canals sense head movements but do not give any information about the movement of other parts of the body.

Information Routes

A signal begins when the cilia on a hair cell are sheared by gravity or acceleration. This causes secretion of a neurotransmitter (a chemical). The electrical signal created by the neurotransmitter travels in a neuron (nerve cell) along the vestibulo-cochlear nerve to the brain.

This sensory information goes directly to at least two areas of the brain: the vestibular nuclear complex and the cerebellum. Most of the balance information goes to the vestibular nuclear complex, also called the vestibular nuclei. As explained below, these are way stations for the information.

The vestibular nuclear complex (VNC) is found in the brainstem of the brain.

The brainstem is the lower part of the brain that includes the medulla, pons, and mesencephalon. This brain area is important because it regulates automatic (autonomic) functions, such as breathing, heart beat, blood pressure, eye movements, the gastrointestinal tract, and balance. It represents the highway through which information arrives and leaves the cortex of the brain.

The VNC receives all the vestibular information coming to the brain and sends it to places needing the information. It sends movement (motor) commands to the muscles of the eyes, neck, chest, arms, and legs. It probably sends information to the autonomic nervous system for use in maintaining blood pressure and selecting breathing muscles. Vestibular information is also passed directly to the cerebellum, then returns to the VNC in a feedback configuration. From the VNC and cerebellum, information is sent to the cortex through the thalamus.

In depth: The vestibulo-cochlear nerve (eighth cranial nerve) contains tens of thousands of nerve fibers serving the inner ear. Generally speaking, the vestibular branch contains vestibular fibers, and the cochlear branch contains cochlear fibers. The fibers originate in the various organs of the inner ear, but at their exit converge in two major nerves—auditory and vestibular— then run together to the brain in the eighth nerve.

While studying the vestibulo-cochlear nerve carefully in 1940, A.T. Rasmussen found that a separation does not always exist between the vestibular and cochlear branches and that sometimes vestibular nerve fibers overlap with cochlear fibers. Figure 4-1 shows a cross-section of the vestibulo-cochlear nerve with vestibular fibers embedded in the cochlear part of the nerve. This means that if the vestibular branch were intentionally cut to stop vertigo, vestibular fibers might be left behind. The degree of fiber overlap would depend on where the cut was made, either closer to or further from the brain. The place where it is cut depends on the surgical procedure selected by the surgeon.

In Rasmussen's own words, "In [the figure], nearly one-fifth of the apparent cochlear nerve is occupied by vestibular fibres. In surgical resection of what is presumably the vestibular nerve, about one-fourth of the vestibular fibres in this case would escape being cut."

Figure 4-1: Fiber overlap. In this illustration, the vestibulo-cochlear nerve is represented by two distinct trunks, one of which is apparently purely vestibular (darker stippling), while the other is mostly cochlear but with a prominent vestibular region amounting to about one-fifth of the cross-sectional area of the trunk. Cutting the vestibular trunk would not cut all the vestibular fibers. (From Rasmussen, A. T., "Studies of the VIIIth Cranial Nerve of Man," *Laryngoscope*, 50:67-83, 1940, with permission from Lippincott-Raven Publishers.)

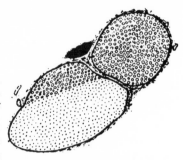

Using Vestibular Information

The movement and gravity information collected by the inner ear is used for more than balance. It is also used for clear vision, a steady head, and some of the body's automatic functions. The majority of this information is used immediately and reflexively by the vestibular nuclear complex of the brain. It does this through the use of several vestibular reflexes including the vestibulo-ocular reflex, vestibulo-collic reflex, vestibular autonomic reflexes, and the vestibulo-spinal reflex.

Clear Vision

Vision and the vestibular system work together to enhance visual accuracy. The vestibulo-ocular reflex (VOR) uses vestibular information to reposition the eyes during movement involving the head. This repositioning keeps the eyes fixed on whatever you are looking at. If your eyes did not move appropriately, things in your field of vision would appear to bounce. More information about the VOR and vision can be found in Chapter 5, "Vision."

Another vestibular reflex, the vestibulo-collic reflex (VCR), also helps to keep your eyes directed at whatever you are looking at by positioning your head rapidly using movement and gravity information.

Steady Head

The vestibulo-collic reflex (VCR) keeps your head steady and in an appropriate position, usually vertical.

Autonomic Adjustments

A number of automatic body functions, including blood pressure and breathing, are regulated by the autonomic nervous system (ANS). The ANS uses vestibular information to institute immediate changes in these body functions to maintain a normal or healthy internal environment.

For example, if no immediate changes in blood vessel diameter occurred when you stood up, your blood pressure would drop, and the amount of blood getting to vital organs, such as your brain, would be inadequate. This could cause lightheadedness or possibly a temporary loss of consciousness.

Position changes can also automatically affect breathing. There is evidence that position changes result in increased depth and frequency of respirations, change in the diaphragm, and changes in some of the chest muscles. These changes may occur via a vestibulo-phrenic reflex. (The phrenic nerve serves the diaphragm.)

Note: An entire book is available about this topic: Yates, B.J. and Miller, S.D. *Vestibular Autonomic Regulation.* Boca Raton, Florida: CRC Press, Inc., 1996.

Balance

Vestibular information is used for all the muscle changes or adjustments necessary to stay upright and move around safely. The vestibular branch of the vestibulo-cochlear nerve sends vestibular information to the vestibular nuclear complex, which sends movement commands down the spinal cord to muscles in the neck, trunk, arms, and legs via the vestibulo-spinal reflex (VSR) and the VCR.

Definition: Balance is defined by *Stedman's Medical Dictionary* as a state of repose between two or more antagonistic forces that exactly counteract each other. With relation to human balance, this generally means using your muscles to counteract gravity and other forces by keeping your center of gravity aligned properly over your feet.

Balance is much more complicated than hearing. Why?

1. Balance is maintained only if the appropriate information is collected and the body is able to make necessary muscle changes.

2. Much of balancing occurs without our conscious knowledge or participation. This makes it difficult to describe normal and abnormal balance sensation and function.

3. Your balance can't be maintained with inner ear vestibular information alone. For proper balance, your brain must also receive information from two other sensory systems—vision and proprioception. Several conditions must be met, and your body must make

appropriate muscle changes to compensate for differences in height, weight, and practice.

Table 4-1: Conditions That Must Be Met
Before Normal Balance Can Occur

- Your inner ears must be functioning normally.
- Your brain (cerebrum, cerebellum, brainstem) must be functioning properly.
- You must be awake and alert.
- Your spinal cord must be working.
- Your muscle strength must be adequate, especially the leg and trunk muscles.
- Your joints must have adequate flexibility, particularly the ankles, knees, and hips.

Systems Involved in Balance

Ideally, three different sensory systems—the vestibular, the visual, and the proprioceptive (also sometimes called the somatosensory)—collect the information needed for balance.

Vision contributes quite a bit to balance. It helps you to avoid obstacles. With vision, you can tell if only your head is moving or if the movement includes your entire body. Constant movement, not sensed by the vestibular apparatus, can be detected with vision. The direction and speed of movement can be seen. Vision can help determine where vertical and horizontal are and if you are "straight" or leaning to the side.

Definition: Proprioception is the information about gravity, position, surfaces, and stretch and motion of the muscles and joints that is collected by the system of pressure sensors scattered around the skeletal muscles, tendons, joints, ligaments, and connective tissue covering the bones and muscles. This information is used to determine what movement is being undertaken and where different body parts are in relationship to one another. You need proprioception to find the tip of your nose with your finger when your eyes are closed, for example.

Proprioception also contributes a lot of necessary information for balance. This system senses the stress in the muscles. During standing, the stress is caused by the force of gravity, which will pull your weight to the ground if your muscles do not contract. Some of the most important proprioceptors are in the neck. These neck receptors give the brain the input needed to determine if only the head is moving or if the movement sensed by the vestibular apparatus is caused by movement of the entire body.

Vision and proprioception supply information the vestibular apparatus is unable to get, and they also collect partially duplicated information. Thus the "system" for collecting balance information is redundant when all three systems are working properly.

Because of the redundancy or duplication of information, with practice you can stand upright and walk without vestibular input if you are not in a visually confusing situation and you are walking on a firm surface.

Successful balance ability, when you are up and about, depends upon how you are able to use your muscles during different situations. The way your brain responds to situations requiring adjustments to maintain balance depends not only on the information collected by the inner ears and other sensory inputs but also on your muscles and their attached nerves. Your motor (movement) response to changing situations depends upon your expectations, experience, and practice.

When you know what to expect, your brain is better able to make the necessary adjustments. For example, if you are subjected to several series of identical changes, you learn what to expect and make rapid and accurate adjustments. If, on the other hand, you are subjected to a series of random changes, your adjustments will not be as rapid or accurate.

Experience with different situations is also something that can enhance balance. For example, your first few attempts at riding a bicycle were probably not successful. At some point you "got it," that is, you experienced a moment of balance on two wheels, and after that you "understood" what you needed to do. This kind of knowledge cannot be gained by watching someone else ride a bicycle or by being told what two-wheeled riding is like. Once you experience balance under cycling conditions, you keep the experience in your brain, and you can revisit it even after years of not riding a bicycle. Returning to a bicycle after years of being away is easy compared to learning to ride the first time.

Practice, performing an activity over and over, improves balance in that activity and usually results in improvement. For example, trying to change the swing of an experienced baseball player or golfer will usually result initially in a slow, stiff, uneasy swing. With many repetitions, the swing will feel and look natural (and may improve the batting average or golf score).

Vestibular Damage

Changes and damage can occur from Meniere's disease in the vestibule and semicircular canals of the inner ear. The original

English language description of endolymphatic hydrops by Hallpike and Cairns describes changes in all three areas of the inner ear: cochlea, vestibule, and semicircular canals.

As in the cochlea, the membranous labyrinth (endolymph-filled space) of the vestibule and semicircular canals presumably becomes enlarged because of an increase of endolymph amount (volume). This enlargement can actually increase to the point that the membranous labyrinth totally occupies the space meant for perilymph.

The vestibular damage and changes that can occur in endolymphatic hydrops include utricular and saccular enlargement, ruptured semicircular canal walls (the membranous labyrinth), abnormal collections of blood, hair cell disintegration, lifting of the otolithic membrane, and chemical environment changes.

All parts of the vestibular apparatus can sustain damage from endolymphatic hydrops, and this can lead to temporary or permanent problems with equilibrium, eye movement, neck movement, and body movement.

References

_____. *Stedman's Medical Dictionary*. 25th edition. Baltimore: Williams and Wilkins, 1990.

Alexander, N.B. "Postural Control in Older Adults." *Journal of the American Geriatric Society*, 42(1):93-108, 1994.

Baloh, R.W., and Honrubia, V. *Clinical Neurophysiology of the Vestibular System*. 2nd edition. Philadelphia: F.A. Davis Company, 1990.

Bernat, J.L., and Vincent, F.M. *Neurology: Problems in Primary Care*. Los Angeles: PMIC, 1993.

Berne, R.M., and Levy, M.N. *Physiology*. Third edition. St Louis: Mosby-Yearbook, 1993.

Cohen, J., and Keshner, E.A. "Current Concepts of the Vestibular System Reviewed: 2. Visual/Vestibular Interaction and Spatial Orientation." *American Journal of Occupational Therapy*, 43:331-337, 1989.

Guyton, A.C., and Hall, J.E. *Textbook of Medical Physiology*. Philadelphia: W.B. Saunders Company, 1996.

Hallpike, C.S., and Cairns, H. "Observations on the Pathology of Meniere's Syndrome." *Journal of Laryngology and Otology*, 53:625-55, 1938.

Horak, F.B., Shupert, C.L., and Mirka, A. "Components of Postural Dyscontrol in the Elderly: A Review." *Neurobiology of Aging,* 10:727-738, 1989.

Keshner, E.A., and Cohen, H. "Current Concepts of the Vestibular System Reviewed: 1. The Role of the Vestibulospinal System in Postural Control." *American Journal of Occupational Therapy,* 43:331-337, 1989.

Marieb, E.N. *Human Anatomy and Physiology.* Third edition. Redwood City, CA: The Benjamin/Cummings Publishing Company, 1995.

Mira, E. "General View of Vestibular Disorders." *Acta Otolaryn-gologica, Supplement,* 519:13-16, 1995.

Rahn, J.E. *Ears, Hearing, and Balance.* New York: Atheneum, 1984.

Rasmussen, A.T. "Studies of the VIIIth Cranial Nerve of Man." *Laryngoscope,* 50:67-83, 1940.

Schmidt, R.F., and Thews, G. *Human Physiology.* New York: Springer-Verlag, 1989.

Tortora, G.J., and Grabowski, R. *Principles of Anatomy and Physiology.* Seventh edition. New York: Harper Collins College Publishers, 1993.

Wilson, V.J., Boyle, R., Fukushima, K., Rose, P.K., Shinoda, Y., Sugiuchi, Y., and Uchino, Y. "The Vestibulocollic Reflex." *Journal of Vestibular Research,* 5(3):147-170, 1995.

Chapter 5

Vision

As odd as it probably sounds, the eyes are closely linked to the ears, and they depend upon each other for good balance and clear vision. The relationship is a two-way street; the ears help you to see clearly, and the eyes help with your balance. This link is the scientific basis for a good deal of the current, sophisticated vestibular testing like rotary testing, caloric testing (part of an ENG), and computerized dynamic posturography. (For more on these tests, see Chapter 16, "Indirect Vestibular Function Tests.") It is also the reason many people with Meniere's disease experience uncomfortable symptoms that involve vision.

Skeptical? Have you ever watched a movie or TV show and felt as if you were moving? Ever pushed down on the brakes because the car next to yours began to move?

"Being in the aisles looking for what I want and all the while having people moving in all directions around me just makes me so sick I almost run to hurry out of there. I recently saw a neuro-ophthalmologist who told me there is a long medical term for this, but they call it "shopping cart syndrome." He says it's all connected to the problem with my ears. I'm so thankful there really is a name for this and I'm not going crazy. I also can not watch TV and focus on anything that is moving fast across the screen or that has the illusion it is coming at you very fast."
—V.T., Oak Grove, Missouri, letter to the author, 1997

"In 1988 when I was seeing a doctor who specialized in Meniere's I kept telling him how fluorescent lighting hurt my eyes, and it was difficult to keep them opened. Also I had to stop reading as just one line would make my eyes jump and made me dizzy, and nausea would start. I could not move my eyes fast, or vertigo would start. I could not go into a store with a white floor, as the glare from the lights closed my eyes right up. Walking down a grocery store aisle and seeing the stock on the shelves as I walked by made me sick and has put me in vertigo. My doctor told me my eyes have nothing to do with Meniere's. I know they do, as I never had a problem before."
—R.C., Deland, Florida, letter to the author, 1997

Vestibular-Ocular Reflex (VOR)

Nerve cells (neurons) link the inner ears to the eyes. Each hair cell of the vestibular end organs requires only three neurons to link it via other structures to the muscles that move the eyes. This link carries messages and commands from the inner ears to the eyes via the brain.

The movement and gravity information collected by the vestibular areas of the ear are sent to the vestibular area of the brain along the first neuron. Then this information is sent along the second neuron and shared with the brain area that controls eye movement. The third neuron carries commands from the eye movement area of the brain to the muscles attached to the outside of the eye, and the commands cause eye movement. This lightning-quick chain of events is referred to as the vestibulo-ocular reflex or VOR.

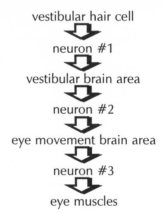

The VOR is different from many reflex systems because it can be modified by the brain. This difference helps to maintain clear vision under the greatest number of conditions but also makes its function more complicated and difficult to explain or understand.

The VOR uses vestibular information to adjust your eyes smoothly in the opposite direction when your head is moved. Not only do the eyes move in a direction precisely opposite to the head movement, but they do so at the same time and at the same speed as the head movement. Without this action, your eyes would be in a fixed position with respect to your head during movements like walking, running, and driving, and the world would appear to be bouncing up and down with each step or bump in the road. The look would be similar to the bouncing picture an inexperienced camera operator might shoot with a video camera.

The "seeing" part of the eye is the retina, located at the back of the eye. To see an object clearly and keep seeing it while you move, the image of the object must be kept still on the back of the eye.

Rotation testing is a convenient way for doctors to determine how well the VOR is working. The speed and timing of the eye movement response are analyzed to determine if they are within the normal range.

Vision and Balance

Balance is not maintained purely by information from the vestibular parts of the inner ear. Two other systems, vision and proprioception, are involved in balance. The best, most efficient balance occurs when all three systems continuously contribute their information to balance. However, if one system is lost, the other two can provide enough information for you to move around within limitations after you practice. Even so, depending on vision or proprioception too much for balance can create new problems.

Vision assists in balance by helping to determine how your body is moving with respect to objects in your environment. For example, if you move forward, objects you are looking at grow larger on your retina, while objects you are moving away from appear to shrink. The problem with primarily using vision for balance is that it is ambiguous and allows the brain to think there is movement when there is none. Busy patterns on carpets, curtains, or wall paper; stripes on a crosswalk (zebra crossing); movement across a TV or movie screen, or just moving the eyes can all increase the ambiguity. Without normal vestibular function, you can be constantly fooled into thinking that either you are moving or that things near you are moving.

An example of being fooled by vision is called a "vection illusion." If you have ever felt as if you were moving because the car next to you was moving, you have experienced vection illusion. This feeling can be so strong that you will suddenly push harder on your car's foot brake even though you were already braking. This is a "normal" experience if it lasts only a second or so in an otherwise normal environment.

Eye and Vision Problems

Eye and vision problems caused by vestibular dysfunction usually fit into one of four categories:
- Abnormal eye movement
- Impaired or absent VOR
- Visually induced nausea, vertigo, and disorientation
- Miscellaneous vision problems

Abnormal Eye Movement

During attacks, Meniere's disease causes nystagmus. Nystagmus is a jerking of the eyes; in Meniere's disease, it is usually a back and forth (horizontal) movement but can also be torsional (turning). Nystagmus occurs because during an attack the vestibular area of the brain receives unequal signals from the two ears without head movement. This movement of the eyes during an attack is often associated with a sensation of spinning or moving in some way.

Nystagmus is the only eye movement change caused by Meniere's disease that can be seen and measured objectively. Unfortunately, nystagmus can also be present from many things other than Meniere's disease such as other vestibular problems, alcohol intoxication, and brain diseases. If nystagmus is the only sign and there are no other symptoms or clues about its origin, it cannot, on its own, be used to diagnose Meniere's disease.

When nystagmus occurs with the eyes open, objects in the room may appear to jump. It is common to see false movement in the visual periphery (off to the side). Many people who experience nystagmus perceive that something is moving quickly past them, like a fly or a bird.

During the caloric testing section of the ENG (as described in Chapter 16, "Indirect Vestibular Function Tests"), nystagmus is intentionally induced to study inner ear function. At the end of each part of the test, you are instructed to open your eyes and stare at a dot on the ceiling. Staring at that dot is referred to as "visual fixation." In an otherwise normal person, visual fixation can overcome the nystagmus and vertigo caused by the test. Sometimes, people with Meniere's disease can use visual fixation to partly suppress the nystagmus and vertigo of a Meniere's attack.

Impaired or Absent VOR

If your Meniere's disease is severe enough to permanently damage your inner ear or if it is bilateral (affecting both ears), your VOR will likely be abnormal. When your VOR is not working well, your eyes don't automatically adjust their position, and objects in the environment may seem to bounce or blur when you move your head. If you move your head up and down as if nodding your head to mean "yes," objects will bounce up and down. When you move your head from side-to-side (a "no" motion in the U.S.), it will cause odd movement of the environment in those directions. This bouncing and blurring of the vision can make it impossible to recognize the faces of people around you or to read signs while you are walking or otherwise in motion.

This movement of things in the environment caused by a poorly functioning vestibular system in turn makes balance more difficult because it is harder to use vision to determine whether you or objects in your environment are moving.

This bouncing of the vision is called oscillopsia. (Some doctors also may refer to it as Dandy's syndrome.) Oscillopsia is uncommon in people with Meniere's disease. If you experience oscillopsia, you should report it to your doctor, who may be able to "measure" it using dynamic visual acuity tests.

The following is a description of oscillopsia by John Crawford, a physician who lost vestibular function in both ears. Dr. Crawford did not have Meniere's disease, but oscillopsia associated with permanent bilateral loss of vestibular function related to Meniere's disease would presumably be experienced in the same way.

"Most of us have experimented with motion pictures at home. This experience can be used to illustrate the sensations of the patient with motion damage to the vestibular apparatus. Imagine the result of a sequence taken by pointing the camera straight ahead, holding it against the chest and walking at a normal pace down a city street. In a sequence thus taken and viewed on the screen, the street seems to career crazily in all directions, faces of approaching persons become blurred and unrecognizable, and the viewer may even experience a feeling of dizziness or nausea."

Dr. Crawford goes on to recount how his body slowly adapted to this loss and how he was able to resume his career and social activities. He also was able to play doubles tennis. (For more on this kind of adaptation, see Chapter 31, "Compensation.")

Visually-Induced Symptoms

"This winter I had a chance to walk inside a very large lens that had been used on the top of an old lighthouse. It was like walking into a kaleidoscope. You could see through it, but there was no color or movement. The glass was arranged in many different patterns, and it took less than 10 seconds for me to be completely unbalanced. My husband was not bothered at all. After leaving, it took me about 15 minutes to feel normal again."
—A.M., Teaneck, N.J., letter to the author, 1997

When they have problems with the vestibular system, most people will automatically rely more on vision to maintain balance. When you rely more on vision, you are apt to have more movement illusions than normal. When your surroundings appear to be moving or when you move your eyes, you may feel *you* are moving. This can cause nausea, disorientation, and/or vertigo. This is not an "attack" of Meniere's disease, but it can be almost as uncomfortable. These visually stimulated feelings are common in the days after an attack.

If you continue to rely disproportionately on vision during a remission from the attacks of Meniere's disease, visually stimulated symptoms can become a constant companion.

This problem can be treated successfully in many people through vestibular rehabilitation. The aim of this treatment is to discourage such heavy dependence upon vision and promote more use of vestibular information and proprioception through the use of special exercises done several times each day.

Reported Vision Problems

Not everyone with Meniere's disease has visually induced symptoms or trouble with eye movement control, but many do. The problems in Table 5-1 have been reported frequently by people with vestibular disorders such as Meniere's disease.

Table 5-1: Vision Problems Often Reported By People With Vestibular Disorders*
• Blurred vision
• Poor depth perception
• Difficulty reading
• Night blindness
• Trouble tolerating glare
• Discomfort when focusing, particularly on distant objects or scenes
• Lights that seem to glow or emit rays
• Trouble in environments with fluorescent light
• General feeling that the vision is somehow "not right"
• Trouble in environments with flashing lights of any sort
*May or may not be related to the vestibular disorder

"Everything I looked at had tracers or shadows after it. Everything was extra bright to me as if my eyes were dilated."
—A.R., letter to the author, 1997

Medication Effects

Medications used to treat Meniere's disease can also be a cause of difficulty with the eyes or vision.

Drugs such as meclizine and especially scopolamine used to temporarily block vestibular symptoms can cause blurred vision. If you experience blurred vision only after taking these drugs, there's a chance the problem is from the drugs rather than the Meniere's disease.

The antihistamine and anti-anxiety drugs often given to people with Meniere's disease can, at times, cause an increase in nystagmus and oscillopsia because of the sedative effect they have on the brain.

Occasionally, a previously undiagnosed case of glaucoma is discovered when eye pain begins after someone takes drugs for Meniere's disease. If you experience eye pain, particularly when it is not associated with bright light, report it to your doctor's office.

For more details on the side effects of medications used to treat Meniere's disease, see Chapters 21 through 26.

Unrelated Eye Changes

Although a close relationship exists between the vestibular system and the control of eye movement, the broad majority of visual problems have nothing to do with the ears or balance. No eye diseases, including glaucoma, cataracts, and macular degeneration, are known to be associated with Meniere's disease. Table 5-2 lists eye problems unrelated to Meniere's disease.

Table 5-2: Eye Changes Unrelated To Meniere's Disease

- Redness/inflammation
- Swelling of the eyes or eyelids
- Bloodshot eyes
- Itching
- Draining
- Pus
- Eye pupils of unequal size
- Eye pain (when not in bright light)
- Excessive watering
- Drooping eyelid(s)
- Twitching eyelids
- Inability to open or close eyelids
- Any missing vision, including the central and peripheral visual fields
- Crossed eyes

What Helps?

You can try many things to limit the visual problems that can occur with Meniere's disease.

Glare Sensitivity

Dark glasses can reduce the amount of light hitting the eyes. However, never wear dark glasses if you have problems with the headlights of oncoming cars while driving at night.

"For the first year I wore non-prescription glasses with a tint to them to cut down the unbearable glare."
—A.R., letter to the author, 1997

Nystagmus

Some people can slow down or stop their nystagmus during an attack through visual fixation, which means staring or fixing the vision on some unmoving object. If you can't tolerate keeping your eyes open during an attack, try to visualize the presence of an object straight ahead, and stare at it.

"There are two rules for me: one, never close your eyes, and two, pick out something in the room and stare at it without moving your eyes. Since I can't focus, I usually find something easy to spot, but not too large, maybe five feet in front of me."
—A.M., Teaneck, New Jersey, letter to the author, 1997

Visually-Induced Symptoms

Changing your lighting arrangements may help reduce visually-induced symptoms.

"If you must work in an area with fluorescent lights, try lighting your desk or work area with a small incandescent light (the 'regular' type electric bulb)."
—"Fuzzy Vision," VEDA flyer, 1992

The following advice applies to vestibular problems in general, but it is good advice also for people in the later stages of Meniere's disease or for whom long periods of time pass between attacks and who have constant visual or visually stimulated symptoms.

"Exposing yourself cautiously and incrementally to provoking environments can speed the adaptation process. If long periods pass between your attacks and you have constant visually stimulated symptoms, staying at home, lying down (perhaps in a dark room) will almost certainly prevent adaptation."
—"Fuzzy Vision," VEDA flyer, 1992

Safety Tips

Steps to protect your eyes and vision can be found in Chapter 34, "Preservation, Protection."

Major Concepts

- Inner ear function is related to clear vision during head movements.

- Some types of visual difficulties are common in Meniere's disease.

- Visual problems lingering weeks and months after the last attack of Meniere's may be treatable.

- Nausea and vertigo induced by visual stimuli are not an "attack" of Meniere's disease.

References

_____. *Taber's Cyclopedic Medical Dictionary,* 15th edition. Philadelphia: F.A. Davis Co., 1985.

Jacobson, G.P., Newman, C.W., and Kartush, J.M. *Handbook of Balance Function Testing,* St. Louis: Mosby Year Book, 1993.

Sharpe, J.A., and Barber, H.O. *The Vestibulo-Ocular Reflex and Vertigo.* New York: Raven Press, 1993.

Shupert, C.L. "Fuzzy Vision." Vestibular Disorders Association flyer, 1992.

Chapter 6

Possible Causes

T he cause of Meniere's disease is unknown. However, many theories have been proposed to explain the symptoms or things that might aggravate them. Listed here in alphabetical order, these things have included abnormal circulation, adrenal-pituitary insufficiency, allergy, autoimmune disease, autonomic nervous system malfunction, bacterial infection, blockage of endolymph, estrogen insufficiency, head injury, heredity, hormonal imbalance, malformed or small endolymphatic sac, malfunction in the use of foods by the body (high cholesterol, triglycerides, or lipids), meningitis, menstrual or premenstrual problems, noise pollution (noise trauma or acoustic trauma), otosclerosis, stress, and viral infection.

Possible Causes of Attack Symptoms

The specific events occurring inside the inner ear that cause the awful symptoms of a Meniere's attack are not known. The most widely-accepted theories are:

- Increased endolymph pressure causes ruptures within the membranous labyrinth that allow endolymph and perilymph to mix and cause the symptoms. When the ruptures close, the symptoms stop. Alternatively (though this may sound strange), when the ruptures close, the symptoms occur.
- The endolymphatic sac chemical responsible for drawing excess endolymph into the sac starts to be secreted intermittently. When this occurs in someone with hydrops, the intermittent secretion causes an occasional backflow of endolymph into the semicircular canals and cochlea. This stimulates the hair cells and causes vertigo, decreased hearing, and increased tinnitus.
- The presence of excess endolymph pressure alone causes the symptoms. When the amount of endolymph decreases, the symptoms stop.
- A rapid increase in fluid pressure causes periods of asphyxia (no oxygen arriving at the structure) to the structures containing the hair cells.
- An increase in the blood level of a chemical called p-ADH causes a temporary increase in the production of endolymph.

Possible Aggravating Factors

Many theories and ideas exist about factors that might aggravate an attack or make one more likely. Sodium, sugar, caffeine, chocolate, alcohol, fluid retention during the pre-menstrual period, cigarettes, elevated cholesterol, and elevated triglyceride levels, weather or pressure changes, physical and/or mental fatigue, insomnia, and stress have all been blamed.

Almost any condition or situation that can result in fluctuating body fluid levels has been suggested as possibly involved in attacks of Meniere's disease. Examples of this include eating too much salt or sugar (simple carbohydrates), pre-menstrual "bloating," and drinking alcohol.

Food and drink, such as chocolate and coffee, which contain substances capable of changing the blood supply to the inner ear, have also been named as possible factors. Nicotine and elevated cholesterol and/or high triglyceride levels might also affect the blood supply.

Many people with Meniere's disease say they are affected during times of pressure change such as when a weather front moves through. The reason for this is not well understood, but European studies have shown that a pressure change intentionally applied to the ears of someone with Meniere's disease can improve hearing in some people.

> "I was interested to read in the last newsletter that one member found his problems got worse at times of low pressure. . . . This recent spell of high pressure has set me going again!"
> —P.C., *Spin*, Autumn 1995

Non-Attack Symptoms

The "attack" symptoms in Meniere's disease are thought to come from an acute event occurring in the inner ear. Other symptoms caused by temporary and/or permanent damage to the vestibular areas of the inner ear can also occur. These symptoms and their causes are not specific to Meniere's disease. They can be similar for anyone with a damaged vestibular system.

Symptoms such as a feeling of unsteadiness, floating, or falling can occur when someone with a damaged vestibular system walks on a soft surface like a deep rug or beach sand. Or you may have problems with other movements such as bending over, tilting your head backwards, looking at a computer screen, being in a room with flickering or blinking lights, moving your eyes, watching something that is moving, walking down an aisle at the grocery store, moving your head rapidly in any direction, moving your eyes and your head simultaneously, looking at a ceiling fan, trying to maneuver in the dark or in low light conditions, or riding in the back seat of a moving car or other vehicle.

Why do these symptoms occur? When the vestibular areas of the inner ear are not sending signals to the brain or the signals they are sending don't make sense, the brain begins to rely more on vision and proprioception. It is much easier for your brain to be fooled when it uses only two of its usual three sources of balance information. You sense things like unsteadiness, floating, falling, and vertigo when your brain is confused by what you see or feel. Also, as your brain adjusts to the changed level of vestibular information, head movement may not feel right at times.

Other Conditions

Specific conditions are known or thought to sometimes cause symptoms like those of Meniere's disease. This occurs either because the conditions affect the inner ear directly or cause symptoms by acting on the vestibulo-cochlear nerve or the brain. These conditions include syphilis (otosyphilis), Cogan's syndrome, autoimmune inner ear disease, dysautonomia, migraine, perilymph fistula, multiple sclerosis, acoustic neuroma (also called vestibular schwannoma), hypothyroidism, and hyperthyroidism.

Perhaps because of the recent focus on AIDS, syphilis is not spoken or written about much these days, but it has not disappeared. In its later stages, syphilis can affect the inner ear directly and look at times just like Meniere's disease. Syphilis can be diagnosed with a specific blood test and in some cases can be eradicated with appropriate drug therapy.

Cogan's syndrome and autoimmune inner ear disease are both diseases in which the body attacks itself. In the case of Cogan's syndrome, the eyes and many other body structures can also become involved. The autoimmune inner ear disease does not reach beyond the ear and differs from Meniere's disease because it will often affect both ears in rapid succession and is associated with massive and sometimes swift hearing loss along with the other symptoms of ear damage.

Dysautonomia is a dysfunction of the autonomic nervous system and usually comes to involve much more than the ear. It can include other problems such as low blood pressure and a heart condition called mitral valve prolapse.

Migraine is also thought to be capable of causing symptoms similar to those of Meniere's disease. Situations involving migraines and symptoms similar to inner ear symptoms can be complicated. Many people are said to have both Meniere's disease and migraine.

A perilymph fistula is an abnormal opening in the inner ear through which perilymph travels. Sometimes the symptoms are identical to those of Meniere's disease, and at other times they can be quite different. Often neither the diagnosis nor the treatment are simple.

Multiple sclerosis is a disease of the nervous system that on very rare occasion can begin with symptoms like those of Meniere's disease.

An acoustic neuroma is a tumor of the balance nerve and, rarely, the hearing nerve. This rarely causes fluctuating hearing loss and episodes of vertigo. The most typical symptom is one-sided hearing loss and no vertigo. It is only mentioned here because some doctors routinely test for it in patients with the symptoms of Meniere's disease.

References

_____. U.K. Meniere's Society. *Spin.* Autumn 1995.

Andrews, J.C., Gregory, A.A., and Honrubia, V. "The Exacerbation of Symptoms in Meniere's Disease During the Premenstrual Period." *Archives of Otolaryngology—Head and Neck Surgery,* 118:74-78, 1992.

Arenberg, I.K. *Surgery of the Inner Ear.* New York: Kugler, 1991.

Bachynski, B., and Wise, J. "Cogan's Syndrome: A Treatable Cause of Neurosensory Deafness." *Canadian Journal of Ophthalmology,* 19(3), 1984.

Baloh, R.W., and Honrubia, V. *Clinical Neurophysiology of the Vestibular System.* Second edition. Philadelphia: F.A. Davis Co., 1990.

Bielory, L., Conti, J., and Frohman, L. "Cogan's Syndrome." *Journal of Allergy and Clinical Immunology,* 85(4):808-815, 1990.

Brookler, K.H., and Glen, M.B. "Meniere's Syndrome: An Approach to Therapy." *Ear, Nose, and Throat Journal,* 74(8):534-542, 1995.

Duke, W.W. "Meniere's Syndrome Caused by Allergy." *Journal of the American Medical Association,* 81(26), 2179-2181, 1923.

Grigsby, J.P., and Johnston, C.L. "Depersonalization, Vertigo, and Meniere's Disease." *Psychological Reports,* 64, 527-534, 1989.

Hinchcliffe, R. "Personality Profile in Meniere's Disease." *Journal of Laryngology and Otology,* 81(5):477-481, 1967.

Linstrom, C.J., and Gleich, L.L. "Otosyphilis: Diagnostic and Therapeutic Update." *Journal of Otolaryngology,* 22:401-408, 1993.

Merchant, S.N., Rauch, S.D., and Nadol, J.B. "Meniere's Disease." *European Archives of Otorhinolaryngology,* 252:63-75, 1995.

Mizukoshi, K., Watanabe, Y., Shojaku, H., Ito, M., Ishikawa, M., Aso, S., Asai, M., and Motoshima, H. "Influence of a Cold Front upon the Onset of Meniere's Disease in Toyama, Japan." *Acta Otolaryngologica, Supplement,* 520:412-414, 1995.

Morrison, A.W. "Anticipation in Meniere's Disease." *Journal of Laryngology and Otology,* 109:499-502, 1995.

Nakagawa, H., Ohashi, N., Kanda, K., and Watanabe, Y. "Autonomic Nervous System Disturbance as Etiological Background of Vertigo and Dizziness." *Acta Otolaryngologica, Supplement,* 504:130-133, 1993.

Pappas, D., Crawford, W., and Coughlan, C. "Dizziness and the Autonomic Dysfunction Syndrome." *Otolaryngology—Head and Neck Surgery,* 94:186-194, 1986.

Pappas, D.G., and Banyas, J.B. "A Newly Recognized Etiology of Meniere's Syndrome: A Preliminary Report." *Acta Otolaryngologica, Supplement,* 485:104-107, 1991.

Parker, W. "Meniere's Disease: Etiologic Considerations." *Archives of Otolaryngology—Head and Neck Surgery,* 121:377-382, 1995.

Pfaltz, C.R. *Controversial Aspects of Meniere's Disease.* Stuttgart: Georg Thieme Verlag, 1986.

Rauch, S.D., Merchant, S.N., and Thedinger, B.A. "Meniere's Syndrome and Endolymphatic Hydrops: Double-Blind Temporal Bone Study." *Annals of Otology, Rhinology, and Laryngology,* 98:873-882, 1989.

Schuknecht, H.F. *Pathology of the Ear.* Cambridge, Mass.: Harvard University Press, 1974.

Shea, J.J., Jr. "Classification of Meniere's Disease." *American Journal of Otology,* 14(3):224-229, 1993.

Vollertsen, R.S., McDonald, T.J., Younge, B.R., Banks, P.M., Stanson, A.W., and Ilstrup, D.M. "Cogan's Syndrome: 18 Cases and a Review of the Literature." *Mayo Clinic Proceedings,* 61:344-361, 1986.

Watanbe, Y., Mizukoshi, K., Shojaku, H., Watanabe, I., Hinoki, M., and Kitahara, M. "Epidemiological and Clinical Characteristics of Meniere's Disease in Japan." *Acta Otolaryngologica, Supplement,* 519:206-210, 1995.

Part II:
Symptoms

Crucial to the diagnosis of Meniere's disease, symptoms also help define the Meniere's experience for those who must live it.

Chapter 7

Symptoms

S omeone diagnosed with Meniere's disease will view the symptoms as extremely important; so will the doctor.
Symptoms are particularly important to the doctor because
no test can rule in Meniere's disease and rule out all other inner ear
problems. (For information on tests, see Chapters 13 through 18.)
Instead, symptoms are used to diagnose the condition and to chart its
cyclical and/or progressive changes.

"Most physicians feel that the only true way to diagnose
Meniere's disease is by the symptoms."
—B.W. Blakely, M.D. and M.E. Siegel,
Feeling Dizzy: Understanding and Treating Vertigo,
Dizziness and Other Balance Disorders, 1995

"In 1861 Prosper Meniere described an illness with a unique
constellation of symptoms thought to be due to an abnormality of the inner ear. Today, diagnosing Meniere's disease
still rests on finding these same symptoms and signs."
—J.D. Macias, M.D., *Steady,* 1994

"There has been very little progress made in developing new
methods to specifically diagnose Meniere's disease. The diagnosis is usually made on the basis of the history and the characteristic low tone SHL [sensorineural hearing loss]."
—J.S. Brown, *Laryngoscope,* 1983

The American Academy of Otolaryngology-Head and Neck Surgery
(the largest specialty organization for doctors treating the ear) has published guidelines for describing treatment results obtained in Meniere's
disease. The presence of the four major symptoms of Meniere's—
recurrent, spontaneous, episodic vertigo; hearing loss; aural fullness,
and **tinnitus**—are the only diagnostic criteria suggested.

The Symptoms

The major symptoms do not usually appear simultaneously.
Years can go by between the appearance of the first and second or
third symptoms. In a 30-year U.S. study, 40.5 percent of the people
diagnosed with Meniere's disease experienced more than a two-year

lapse between the appearance of the first and second symptoms; 37.2 percent had them occur within the first three months, and the remainder had them appear in three to nine months. One Japanese study of 28 people found that only five had all the symptoms at the beginning; six started with vertigo, and 17 began with hearing loss or tinnitus. In a German study involving 574 people, only 27 percent began with all the symptoms.

Unfortunately Meniere's disease can create more than just the four major symptoms. The symptoms of Meniere's can be divided into two groups, the *major symptoms* and the *adjunctive symptoms*. The major symptoms are the group of four used to diagnose the condition. The adjunctive symptoms are all the others that can occur because of Meniere's disease.

Important points: The adjunctive symptoms can be present in many other diseases and conditions of the inner ear and elsewhere; they are not specific to Meniere's disease. Individuals can have only a few or almost all of the symptoms. Some are present only during "attacks," others only after attacks. Some are present during the "remission" between attacks, and some are seen during "late-stage" Meniere's, when the disease has progressed quite far.

The table on the next page lists the symptoms. (We have tried to be as complete as possible in assembling this list, but some may have been omitted.)

Grouping Symptoms

For convenience, we have grouped Meniere's disease symptoms into the following categories:
• the warning before an impending attack
• the attack
• the aftermath of an attack
• the remission between the aftermath and the next attack

These categories refer to the *Meniere's cycle* (warning, attack, aftermath, remission), which can occur again and again in "early-stage" Meniere's.

Many of these symptoms can and do occur during more than one time period. We have grouped these symptoms into the time periods of which they are most typical.

See Tables 7-1 through 7-5 on the facing page and on page 64.

Symptom Stages

The "stages" of Meniere's disease are referred to many times in different reference sources. Unfortunately no universal, agreed-upon method exists for identifying these stages.

Some experts simply say that the early or beginning stages of Meniere's disease are characterized by a fluctuating hearing loss, tinnitus, ear fullness, and episodes of vertigo and that the late or advanced stages of Meniere's consist of a permanent hearing loss

---

Table 7-1: Possible Symptoms of Meniere's Disease

Major Symptoms

aural pressure	tinnitus	vertigo
hearing loss		

Adjunctive Symptoms

anger/rage	groping for stable	poor appetite
anxiety	objects (posts,	poor depth
blurred vision	trees, etc.)	perception
bouncing vision	when walking	queasiness
clumsiness	groping for words	rapid pulse
cold sweat	hangover feeling	seasick feeling
depression	headache	sleepiness
diarrhea	heavy head feeling	slurred speech
difficulty concentrating	intensified glare	sound distortion
difficulty focusing	jerking of vision	sound sensitivity
difficulty reading	lightheadedness	staggering
difficulty turning	(faintness)	stiff neck
difficulty walking	loss of self-confidence	stiffness
in the dark	loss of self-esteem	stumbling
difficulty watching	loss of self-reliance	sudden balance loss
movement	malaise	sudden falls
distractability	motion intolerance	trembling
drunk feeling	motion sickness	unsteadiness
eye jerking	nausea	visual distortions
fatigue	neck ache	vomiting
fear	palpitations	worry

Table 7-2: Possible Warning Symptoms Before an Attack

balance disturbance	increased tinnitus
dizziness	lightheadedness
headache	sound sensitivity
increased ear pressure	vague feeling of uneasiness
increased hearing loss	

Table 7-3: Symptoms Likely During an Attack

aural fullness	fear	rapid pulse
anxiety	hearing loss	tinnitus
blurred vision	jerking of vision	trembling
cold sweat	nausea	vertigo
eye jerking	palpitations	vomiting

Table 7-4: Possible Symptoms of the Aftermath

clumsiness	fatigue	poor appetite
difficulty focusing, especially on distant objects	hangover feeling	seasick feeling
	headache	sleepiness
	heavy head	sound distortion
difficulty reading	lightheadedness	staggering
difficulty turning	, (faintness)	stiff neck
difficulty watching movement	malaise	stiffness
	motion intolerance	stumbling
disequilibrium	motion sick feeling	unsteadiness
distractability	neck ache	visual distortions

Table 7-5: Symptoms Likely During the Remission

anger/rage	loss of self-esteem
a sense of intensified glare from lights	loss of self-confidence
	poor depth perception
fear	poor memory
groping for words	sound sensitivity
loss of self-reliance	worry

(possibly severe), tinnitus, possible ear pressure, and few or no attacks of vertigo. Instead of few or no attacks of vertigo, there may be constant unsteadiness.

Other experts name three auditory stages: (1) the stage of reversible hearing loss, (2) the stage of established fluctuating hearing loss, and (3) the stage of permanent, non-fluctuating hearing loss.

The Committee on Hearing and Equilibrium defines four stages with differing amounts of hearing loss. Stage one has the least amount of hearing loss, and stage four has the most, a profound loss.

In 1993, J. J. Shea in the *American Journal of Otology* suggested the following stages: (1) ear fullness, tinnitus, fluctuating hearing loss, (2) ear fullness, tinnitus, fluctuating hearing loss, and "dizzy spells," (3) ear fullness, tinnitus, increased and permanent hearing loss, and "dizzy spells," (4) ear fullness, tinnitus, increased and permanent hearing loss, no "dizzy spells," and constant unsteadiness especially in darkness, and (5) decreased fullness and tinnitus, pro-

Table 7-6: Possible Symptoms of Late-Stage Meniere's Disease	
a need to look down while walking	difficulty looking through binoculars, cameras,
a need to touch things while walking	microscopes, telescopes, and the like
bouncing vision	significant hearing loss
difficulty walking in the dark	sudden loss of balance
disequilibrium	

found hearing loss, no "dizzy spells," and constant unsteadiness especially in darkness.

In this book we use the terms "early-stage Meniere's" and "late-stage Meniere's" to describe, in a general way, the stages of this progressive disease. In addition, we use the term "Meniere's cycle" and its four components, "warning," "attack," "aftermath," and "remission," to describe symptom groups likely to occur again and again during early-stage Meniere's.

The following five chapters correspond to Tables 7-2 through 7-6 and will give you more information about the warning, the attack, the aftermath, the remission, and late-stage Meniere's disease.

References

Blakely, B.W., and Siegel, M.E. *Feeling Dizzy: Understanding and Treating Vertigo, Dizziness, and Other Balance Disorders.* New York: MacMillan, 1995.

Booth, J.B. *Scott-Brown's Otolaryngology-Otology.* Fifth edition. London: Butterworths, 1987.

Brown, J.S. "A Ten Year Statistical Follow-Up of 245 Consecutive Cases of Endolymphatic Shunt and Decompression with 328 Consecutive Cases of Labyrinthectomy." *Laryngoscope*, 93:1419-1424, 1983.

Cawthorne, T.E. "Meniere's Disease." *Annals of Otolaryngology—Head and Neck Surgery*, 58:18-37, 1947.

Committee on Hearing and Equilibrium. "Committee on Hearing and Equilibrium Guidelines for the Diagnosis and Evaluation of Therapy in Meniere's Disease." *Otolaryngology—Head and Neck Surgery*, 113(3):181-185, 1995.

Haid, C.T., Watermeier, D., Wolf, S.R., and Berg, M. "Clinical Survey of Meniere's Disease: 574 Cases." *Acta Otolaryngologica, Supplement*, 520, 251-255, 1995.

Macias, J.D. "Diagnosing Meniere's Disease." *Steady* (quarterly newsletter of the Meniere's Network), 5(5):1, 1994.

Shea, J.J. "Classification of Meniere's Disease." *American Journal of Otology*, 14(3):224-229, 1993.

Tokumasu, K., Fujino, A., Naganuma, H., Hoshino, I., and Arai, M. "Initial Symptoms and Retrospective Evaluation of Prognosis in Meniere's Disease." *Acta Otolaryngologica, Supplement*, 524, 1996.

Vesterhauge, S. "Meniere's: An Ear Disease." Copenhagen: Danish Meniere's Association, 1996.

Wladislavosky-Waserman, P., Facer, G.W., Kurland, L.T., and Mokri, B. "Meniere's Disease: A 30-Year Epidemiologic and Clinical Study in Rochester, Minn., 1951-1980." *Laryngoscope*, 94:1098-1102, 1984.

Chapter 8
Warning

Some people, perhaps as many as 50 percent, experience symptoms or sensations immediately before an attack phase of Meniere's disease. This experience is commonly called an aura. An aura consists of the symptoms and sensations felt before a sudden, repetitive attack of something. "Aura" is used not only in association with Meniere's disease but to describe the symptoms and sensations that precede a migraine headache or an epileptic seizure. To avoid confusion with migraine or epilepsy, we use the word "warning" instead of aura.

During a Meniere's attack warning, you may experience hearing loss or increased hearing loss, tinnitus or increased tinnitus or a change in the character of the tinnitus, aural pressure or increased pressure, headache, lightheadedness, slight balance disturbance, increased sensitivity to sound, and/or a vague feeling of uneasiness— alone or in any combination. Some people simply say they feel an attack coming on and cannot describe exactly what they feel. In some people, these symptoms continue into the attack and possibly into the aftermath.

> "We were out that evening with friends, I became strangely anxious. By the time we got home I was so dizzy I could hardly get out of the car."
>
> —Jan Morris, *RN*, 1990

A Meniere's attack warning would not be something visual such as a flash of light, spots, or sudden darkness. It would not be a smell, inability to swallow or speak, muscle weakness, or a "blinding" headache, nor would it be any alteration of consciousness such as fainting.

If you experience a warning before an attack, you can use it to get ready. If driving, you can pull over to the side of the road. If at home, you can turn off the oven and make other preparations before the vertigo starts. (For more information on precautions, see Chapter 32, "Coping," and Chapter 33, "Safety.")

References

Cawthorne, T.E. "Meniere's Disease." *Annals of Otolaryngology— Head and Neck Surgery*, 58:18-37, 1947.

Cleveland, P.J., and Morris, J. "Meniere's Disease: The Inner Ear Out of Balance." *RN*, 54:28-32, 1990.

Merchant, S.N., Rauch, S.D., and Nadol, J.B. "Meniere's Disease." *European Archives of Otorhinolaryngology*, 252:63-75, 1995.

Pfaltz, C.R. *Controversial Aspects of Meniere's Disease*. New York: Thieme, Inc., 1986.

Chapter 9
Attack

The "attack" refers to symptoms occurring when a physical change, not fully understood, takes place within the inner ear and produces an episode of perhaps violent, spinning vertigo that may be accompanied by tinnitus, hearing loss, and aural (ear) fullness along with nausea, vomiting, abnormal eye movement, vision disturbances, sweating, rapid heart beat, palpitations, cold sweat, fear, anxiety, trembling, anger, hyperventilation, and blurred vision.

Note: Spinning vertigo could also be described as whirling, circling, rotating, rotational, rotatory, or turning vertigo.

The following is a personal account of an attack:

"Why is the house so quiet I thought, then I realized I couldn't hear. A jet roared inside my head, blocking out all other sounds. Dizziness overcame me. Somehow I made it to the bathroom before the whirlwind inside my head knocked me to the floor. With all the intense pressure and pain inside my ear, I couldn't think. My balance was completely gone. I couldn't even lift my head. I prayed for my family, and made my peace with God."

—Jan Morris, *RN*, 1990

Here are more descriptions from various sources about the experience of an attack of Meniere's disease:

"The only part (of me) that could function was my voice."

—G.H., *Spin*, Spring 1996

"Everything around me was moving and Niagara roared in my left ear. It was as if I was the water in a bucket, being forced to the bottom by some giant who was rapidly swinging the pail in a circle."

—Gertrude Blancher, R.N.,
American Journal of Nursing, 1974

"I did not know until then that such dizziness existed. I had never before been so dizzy that I couldn't stand or walk but could only get down on the floor and crawl to wherever I needed to go. . . ."

—V.G., Oregon, *On The Level*, Fall 1996

"I felt like I was falling into the earth's pit. I clung to my bed's headboard so I would not slip away."

—B.L., California, letter to the author, 1996

". . . dizziness and ringing in the ears like all the bells of Halle, Leipzig, Erfurt and Wittenberg."

—Martin Luther as quoted in the *American Journal of Otology*, 1979

The Major Symptoms

Vertigo

Vertigo is the perception of movement (either of yourself or of objects around you) that is not occurring or is occurring differently from what you perceive. Vertigo is not a fear of heights; it is not trouble with ladders; it is not being lightheaded.

What is it like? The vertigo of Meniere's disease is spontaneous, recurrent, and episodic, and it is usually described as violent spinning.

Spontaneous vertigo is vertigo without an apparent cause. If the spinning always comes when you roll onto your left side, for example, it is not spontaneous. Benign paroxysmal positional vertigo (BPPV), the most common cause of episodic vertigo, is an example of an inner problem that causes non-spontaneous vertigo. If you have BPPV, you may be able to deliberately provoke vertigo by moving your head in a certain way.

Recurrent vertigo is vertigo returning after an absence. Vertigo appearing once and not returning is not recurrent vertigo. Vertigo that comes and stays is also not recurrent.

The vertigo of Meniere's disease comes in an episode, commonly called an attack. It has a starting point and an ending point and lasts minutes to hours. If the spinning lasts more than 24 hours, the problem may not be Meniere's disease. A couple of other vestibular problems, labyrinthitis and vestibular neuronitis, can cause violent vertigo lasting more than 24 hours.

The Meniere's vertigo most likely occurs because of physical change in the inner ear, as described in Chapter 4, "Balance and the Other Vestibular Functions."

Hearing Loss

The hearing loss of Meniere's disease occurs in the problem ear and is sensorineural. It is sometimes referred to as nerve deafness. This loss usually occurs in the lower frequencies (low-pitched sounds) and may occur only during attacks (especially at the beginning of the disease), or it may be present between attacks. The amount of hearing loss has no relationship to the severity of the vertigo. Someone experiencing mild short attacks might have a severe hearing loss, while someone enduring frequent long attacks of vertigo might have almost no hearing loss.

Definition: Sensorineural hearing loss (SNHL) results from damage to the hearing nerve or cochlear hair cells. It is not the result of a problem with the outer or middle ear.

Aural Fullness

Aural fullness can also be called aural pressure, ear pressure, or ear fullness. This is a feeling of fullness or pressure in the ear that can also be described as a "stopped up" feeling or a general feeling of pressure within the head. The fullness may also be described as follows:

". . .my ear felt full and painful . . . ."

—S.D. Farber,
The American Journal of Occupational Therapy, 1989

The number of people with Meniere's disease who have aural fullness is not known. Three studies that addressed this question found that 56 percent (German study), 73 percent (U.S. study) and 22.2 percent (another U.S. study) of the members of the study groups had aural fullness.

Oddly, no nerve capable of transmitting a sense of fullness from the ear to the brain has been discovered. Continuous aural pressure or fullness is difficult to explain if the inner ear cannot send such information to the brain. Assuming that a nerve exists but has not yet been discovered, the pressure can be explained by the presence of endolymphatic hydrops. This overabundance of endolymph can swell the membranous labyrinth throughout the entire inner ear. It can grow to the point that the membranous labyrinth totally occupies the space meant for perilymph.

If everyone with a diagnosis of Meniere's disease has endolymphatic hydrops, why doesn't everyone have fullness? This question remains unanswered.

Tinnitus

Tinnitus is the medical term for what is commonly referred to as "ringing in the ears." The tinnitus of Meniere's disease cannot be heard by anyone but the person experiencing it. It occurs in the "problem" ear. The pitch or frequency is usually low and has been described as sounding like sea shore hissing (most common), bells ringing, crickets chirping, water rushing, roaring, blowing, buzzing, and radio static. It should not sound like a voice or voices. It may be present only during attacks, or it may occur all the time and increase or decrease in intensity during an attack.

In many cases, the tinnitus is very annoying and can be a big discomfort. Here is one description of tinnitus that occurred during an attack of Meniere's disease:

> ". . . Niagara roared in my left ear."
> —Gertrude Blancher, R.N.,
> *American Journal of Nursing,* 1974

Note: Tinnitus occurs in two forms, **subjective** and **objective.** The tinnitus of Meniere's disease is subjective, only heard by the person experiencing it. Objective tinnitus is a rare type that can be heard by other people. If your doctor has put his or her ear next to yours, she or he was probably checking for objective tinnitus.

Tinnitus has received a lot of attention recently, partly because it's such a common problem. Millions of Americans have tinnitus for a multitude of reasons, including noise damage. A great deal of research continues to involve this problem.

In many cases, tinnitus increases as a hearing loss progresses. It's usually the most annoying when it's a new experience and usually becomes less annoying as time goes by.

Adjunctive Symptoms

Nausea and Vomiting

It has been known for a long time that motion such as travel by car, boat, or airplane can cause nausea and vomiting. Meniere's disease and other problems with vestibular function can do the same. The brain's vomiting center actually causes vomiting after receiving information from the inner ear, digestive tract, and/or two other brain areas.

A theory about the value of vomiting to human evolution can be found in an article by K.S. Longbridge in *The Journal of Otolaryngology* in 1983. (See the "Reference" section of this chapter.)

Along with being just plain uncomfortable, nausea and vomiting can be accompanied by a change to a paler skin color, increased amounts of saliva, and hyperventilation. When vomiting goes on long enough, it can cause weakness, dehydration, and imbalance of body minerals (also called electrolytes). This can occur more quickly in small children, people over 65, and in individuals with other serious medical conditions such as diabetes mellitus or heart disease. Determining exactly when to call the doctor about vomiting is difficult, but if the vomiting goes on for more than 12 hours, it is probably time.

Nausea and vomiting can also lead to depression, poor appetite, and loss of morale, particularly when it occurs repeatedly.

Things that can make nausea and/or vomiting worse include movement, anxiety, foods with a high fat content, thinking about previous situations that have caused nausea and/or vomiting, and, possibly, a full bladder.

Cold Sweat and Other Symptoms

Cold sweat, anxiety, trembling, increased heart rate, palpitations, terror, hyperventilation, and blurred vision can be attributed to the autonomic nervous system. It regulates the body's automatic functions such as heart rate, breathing, blood pressure, urine production, pupil size, digestion, release of adrenaline, and sweating.

The autonomic nervous system is also responsible for the "fight or flight" response humans have to danger and stress. This system will "rev up" certain areas of the body so that we can either stand and fight or run as fast as possible out of harm's way. This "rev up" includes an increase in the heart rate, increase in rate and depth of breathing, dilation of the pupils, goose bumps, sweating, release of adrenaline from the adrenal glands, decrease in urine production, decrease in saliva, increased blood flow to certain areas and decreases to others, and a general increase in the metabolic rate (the speed at which the body operates).

This is an excellent response if we are attacked by a dog, for example. It allows us to "hit the ground running." But, if we really are not physically threatened, the autonomic nervous system changes can be not only uncomfortable but actually bad for our general health. These changes can be so uncomfortable and pronounced they seem to be the problem rather than a response. They make the "attack" feel like an extremely serious, body-wide problem rather than "just" an inner ear problem.

"My heart felt like it would pound out of my chest."
—Jan Morris, *RN,*1990.

"It is a terrible feeling of panic and fear, and it's accompanied by a deep sense inside that everything is wrong. . . ."
—C.D., *Barrow*, December 1992

"The symptoms and signs that follow immediately upon an injury to the labyrinth are widespread and are often so terrifying in their intensity that observers unused to the ways of the labyrinth may find it difficult to believe that such a profound disturbance can be caused by injury to such a modest organ. . . ."
—T.E. Cawthorne,
Proceedings of the Royal Society of Medicine, 1945

These symptoms can also take on something of a life of their own. Symptoms that began because of intense vertigo can continue because of the fear, anxiety, increased blood pressure, or increased heart rate. In his book, *Phobia Free*, Harold Levinson, M.D. suggests that this response can continue not only beyond the attack's vertigo but can also occur in separate episodes not involving intense vertigo. Symptoms can be "triggered" by things like worry, fear, anger, and particular body movements, or movements in your field of vision.

Note: *Phobia Free* was written for the general public. It may explain much about these "other" symptoms and their unwanted appearance. For bibliographic details, see the reference section at the end of this chapter.

A relationship also exists between these autonomic nervous system changes and panic attacks. These symptoms are similar to those experienced by people diagnosed with panic disorder. In fact, the similarity has created another controversy. Does a vestibular problem create panic symptoms, or do panic symptoms cause vestibular symptoms such as vertigo? *Phobia Free* deals with this question, as does *Vestibular Autonomic Regulation*, on a smaller scale.

Some people can have a near-attack experience in which they have all these autonomic nervous system symptoms but do not experience vertigo or hearing loss.

"I felt just like I was about to have an attack. My heart was pounding, the sweat was pouring, I felt like my insides were trembling but the spins didn't come."
—P. P., British Columbia, in a letter to the author, 1996

Disturbed Vision

Your eyes can be affected by the vestibular parts of your ears because vestibular information is used to make appropriate eye movements. (See Chapter 5, "Vision.") Eye jerking and blurred vision can occur during an attack. The jerking can be so bad that opening your eyes will cause vomiting. The movement is generally from side to side (horizontal) and is called nystagmus. Nystagmus is usually present during an attack.

Blurring can also occur because your autonomic nervous system causes your pupils to dilate in response to an attack. If you have ever had a full eye examination with pupil dilation, you are familiar with the visual changes dilation can cause.

References

_____. Barrow Neurological Institute. "Life with Meniere's Disease Is a Balancing Act for Physician." *Barrow*. December 1992.

_____. U.K. Meniere's Society. *Spin*. Spring 1996

_____. Vestibular Disorders Association. *On the Level*. Fall 1996.

Arenberg, I.K., Countryman, L.F., Bernstein, L.H., and Shambaugh, G.E. "Van Gogh Has Meniere's Disease and Not Epilepsy." *Journal of the American Medical Association*, 264(4):491-493, 1990.

Blakley, B.W., and Siegel, M.E. *Feeling Dizzy: Understanding and Treating Vertigo, Dizziness and Other Balance Disorders*. New York: MacMillan, 1995.

Blancher, G.C. "My Trip Through the Semicircular Canals." *American Journal of Nursing*, 74(10):1842-1843, 1974.

Cawthorne, T.E. "Meniere's Disease." *Annals of Otolaryngology— Head and Neck Surgery*, 58:18-37, 1947.

Cawthorne, T.E. "Vestibular Injuries." *Proceedings of the Royal Society of Medicine*, 270-273, 1945.

Chalat, N.I. "Who Was Prosper Meniere and Why Am I Still So Dizzy?" *American Journal of Otology*, 1(1):52-56, 1979.

Cleveland, P.J., and Morris, J. "Meniere's Disease: The Inner Ear Out of Balance." *RN*, Aug. 10, 54:28-32, 1990.

Conn, H.F. *Conn's Current Therapy*. Philadelphia: W.B. Saunders Company, 1996.

Farber, S.D. "Living with Meniere's Disease: An Occupational Therapist's Perspective." *American Journal of Occupational Therapy*, 43(5):341-343, 1989.

Gibson, W.P., and Arenberg, I.K. "The Circulation of Endolymph and a New Theory of the Attacks Occurring in Meniere's Disease." *Surgery of the Inner Ear.* New York: Kugler Publications. 1990.

Green, J.D., Blum, D.J., and Harner, S.G. "Longitudinal Follow-Up of Patients with Meniere's Disease." *Otolaryngology Head and Neck Surgery,* 104(6):783-788, 1991.

Haid, C.T., Watermeier, O., Wolf, S.R., and Berg, M. "Clinical Survey of Meniere's Disease." *Acta Otolaryngologica, Supplement,* 520:251-255, 1995.

Hallpike, C.S., and Cairns, H. "Observations on the Pathology of Meniere's Syndrome." *Journal of Laryngology and Otolology,* 53:625-55, 1938.

Hawthorn, J. *Understanding and Management of Nausea and Vomiting.* Oxford: Blackwell Science, 1995.

Katsarkas, A. "Hearing Loss and Vestibular Dysfunction in Meniere's Disease," *Acta Otolaryngologica,* 116:185-188, 1996.

Levinson, H.N., and Carter, S. *Phobia Free.* New York: M Evans, 1986.

Longbridge, K.S. "The Value of Nausea and Vomiting Due to Meniere's Disease—A Theory." *The Journal of Otolaryngology,* 12:403-404, 1983.

Marieb, E.N. *Human Anatomy and Physiology.* Redwood City, Calif.: The Benjamin/Cummings Publishing Company, 1995.

Takedo,T., Kakigi, A., and Saito, H. "Antidiuretic Hormone (ADH) and Endolymphatic Hydrops." *Acta Otolaryngologica, Supplement,* 519: 219-222, 1995.

Tokumasu, K., Fujino, A., Naganuma, H., Hoshino, I., and Arai, M. "Initial Symptoms and Retrospective Evaluation of Prognosis in Meniere's Disease." *Acta Otolaryngologica, Supplement,* 524: 43-49, 1996.

Vesterhauge, S. "Meniere: An Ear Disease" (brochure). Copenhagen: Danish Meniere Association, 1996.

Wladislavosky-Waserman, P., Facer, G.W., Kurland, L.T., and Mokri, B. "Meniere's Disease: A 30-Year Epidemiologic and Clinical Study in Rochester, Minn., 1951-1980." *Laryngoscope,* 94: 1098-1102, 1984.

Yardley, L. *Vertigo and Dizziness.* New York: Routledge, 1994.

Yates, B.J., and Miller, A.D. *Vestibular Autonomic Regulation.* Florida: CRC Press, 1996.

Chapter 10
Aftermath

I f you are lucky, you will have little trouble in the period directly after an attack.

"In many instances, following a sound sleep of several hours, the patient woke little the worse for his attack."
—T.E. Cawthorne,
Annals of Otolaryngology—Head and Neck Surgery, 1947

Unfortunately, not everybody returns immediately to "normal" after an attack. When you try to move or focus your eyes, you may feel new symptoms. They may vary in intensity and number from just feeling a "bit off" and tired to being almost unable to get out of bed, and they can last for days if another attack does not occur. These symptoms can interfere with your normal functioning and dampen your desire to do much of anything.

"I had a little turn in my head this morning which though it did not last above a minute, yet, being of the true sort, has made me weak as a dog all day."
—Jonathan Swift, author of *Gulliver's Travels*,
as quoted in *American Journal of Otology*, 1979.

Why so many different sensations after the attack? Balance is basically unconscious and goes on day after day without much thought. With the attacks, balance becomes conscious, something to be constantly aware of. Not only does balance become conscious, it has been disturbed, and the brain requires a period of time to readjust. We have decided to call this period of time the "aftermath."

The brain expects consistent and meaningful vestibular signals at all times. During the attack, the signals change from the norm and change again when the attack stops. The post-attack messages from inner ear to brain may not be identical to the pre-attack messages; this creates a mismatch among the three systems collecting balance information—vision, proprioception, and the vestibular system—and the expectations of the brain. (The brain expects the three systems to supply the same information they have in the past and at the same rates.)

When conditions change, the brain immediately tries to adapt to the new situation. It struggled to do so during the attack and will continue to do so in the two to three days after the attack. As the vestibular signals become consistent, the brain re-acclimates itself, and the symptoms calm down and usually fade away, at least during the beginning or early stages of Meniere's disease.

This disruption in vestibular signals can cause vertigo, lightheadedness, heavyheadedness, visual problems, stiffness, fatigue, increased need for sleep, a hangover feeling, balance problems when you try to move, and a general feeling of "things just not being right" for a few days after the attack. Sometimes there is also a feeling of "unreality." (A *Star Trek* fan might describe it as a temporal anomaly or a parallel reality.)

The aftermath symptoms fit into a few broad categories: head sensations, general feeling, sound affects, vision, stiffness, and movement. (The sound effects may also be caused by the formation of scar tissue from the membranous labyrinth that attaches like a rubber band to the stapes bone.) Each of these broad categories includes several sensations that might be present right after an attack. In the list below, you will find the broad categories, the sensations, descriptions of the sensations, and possible explanations for their occurrence.

General Feeling

You will probably feel fatigue, sleepiness, malaise, and a "hangover" after an attack. It is not unusual for people to sleep for hours and hours past an attack or to actually fall asleep as an attack is "winding down." It can take a few days for your usual amount of energy to return. These feelings can occur for several reasons, as follows:

• You spend a large amount of energy during an attack, particularly if you have had a large reaction from your autonomic nervous system and/or you were vomiting or retching.

• In the days after the attack, maintaining balance requires more effort while your brain gets re-organized and accustomed to any permanent change and possibly begins to rely more upon vision and proprioception for balance.

• A hearing loss can also require you to struggle to hear things, and this may make you tired.

> "After a session in the bathroom was over, I would crawl to the hallway and fall asleep for several hours."
> —V.G., *On the Level*, Fall, 1996

The hangover feelings can include fatigue, headache, desire to avoid contact with other people, sensitivity to lights and sounds, a queasy stomach, and overreaction when surprised. These sensations can feel similar to an alcohol hangover, which is not surprising because alcohol directly affects the inner ear, and the alcohol hangover, or parts of it, may actually be produced by the inner ear.

The fatigue, malaise, sleepiness, and hangover feeling have been described as "brain fog," fuzziness, being washed out or totally drained, and, in Great Britain, as woolly-headedness.

> "I'm writing this whilst taking time off work to recover from that washed out feeling that often follows an attack of Meniere's." —T.H., *Spin*, Winter, 1995

Poor appetite is also common after an attack and may result from not feeling well, the nausea and vomiting during the attack, lingering nausea and/or a digestive system slowdown caused by the "fight or flight" episode.

Head Sensations

Odd head sensations such as lightheadedness or heavyheadedness are fairly common after an attack and can last a few days. These can be distracting and disturbing and make some people feel that something else even more serious is actually happening.

Lightheadedness may be caused by a disruption of the autonomic nervous system, a blood pressure lower than usual, dehydration from the vomiting during the attack, and/or a disturbance of the gravity sensors (utricle and saccule) of the inner ear.

Heavyheadedness is the feeling of the head being heavier than it ought to be. This sensation may also be caused by a disturbance of the inner ear's gravity sensors.

Sound Effects

Diplacusis, a single tone sounding like two tones, is not uncommon. To check to see if you have diplacusis, try whistling one long tone, and decide if it sounds like one tone or two. Diplacusis can occur because of the difference between the "good" ear and the one affected by Meniere's disease.

Hyperacusis, in which sound seems to be louder than it actually is, is another common problem. It can range from slightly annoying to severe, causing you to avoid sound as much as possible. The cause for this problem is really not understood. This symptom is not limited to people with Meniere's disease.

Another possible Meniere's symptom related to sound is called the Tullio phenomenon. With this problem, sound causes vertigo. The Tullio phenomenon may be caused by an enlarged saccule (large because of the excessive amount of endolymph in the inner ear) being pushed by a middle ear bone.

Sound causes the stapes bone to slip in and out through the oval window. If the saccule has enlarged to the point that it touches the oval window on the inner ear side of this opening, stapes movement can affect it.

The sensation of vertigo in response to sound also occurs with a problem called a perilymph fistula. (With this problem, the movement of the stapes bone probably causes perilymph, the other inner ear fluid, to leak from the oval window.)

Vision/Eyes

Visual difficulties are common during and after an attack of Meniere's disease. These problems include difficulty focusing the eyes, difficulty watching movement, visual distortions, and difficulty reading.

Difficulty focusing the eyes might be caused by a lingering autonomic nervous system effect that caused the pupils of the eyes to be larger than usual. (The pupils must be able to contract, or your eyes can't focus properly). Or the cause might be lingering nystagmus.

Watching movement can trigger nausea and dizziness because the movement seen can be mistaken for body movement. It is confusing when proprioception and the vestibular system say that the body is still, and the eyes say it is moving. This confusion creates unpleasant sensations.

Lingering nystagmus (eye jerking) can feel like eye movement or can cause things to appear to jump, particularly in the periphery (off to the side rather than in the middle).

Difficulty reading can be caused by focusing problems, the illusion of false movement when a line of words is scanned, and lingering nystagmus.

Stiffness/Pain

Muscle stiffness, anywhere from head to toe, and headache are also common in the days after an attack.

Holding your neck rigidly to prevent head movement during an attack can cause neck ache. Also, if vestibular information is faulty or absent, your brain may not have the information it needs to control neck muscles in the usual way. The muscles can become tense and stiff.

Other muscles can also stiffen because of the change in vestibular information that occurred during the attack. This information is used for the reflexes that help you move "naturally." When the information is faulty or absent, the muscles of the arms, legs and trunk can become stiff, and movement no longer feels "right."

"If I turned my head, neck and body to the left as a unit, the symptoms were reduced. I felt like the tin man in the *Wizard of Oz.*"

—S.D. Farber,
American Journal of Occupational Therapy, 1989.

Stomach muscles can also ache from vomiting and dry heaves.

Headaches are not usually considered to be a common feature of Meniere's disease, but they do occur.

"It felt as though someone had hit me over the head with a hammer."

—C.D., *On the Level*, Summer 1993

Headaches can be caused by just plain not feeling well, facial muscle strain from trying to focus your eyes, holding your head rigidly during an attack, and vomiting, which can lead to dehydration.

Movement

In the days following an attack, movement can seem to be an adventure rather than something automatic. Staggering, stumbling, and feeling unsteady are common. You may need to hang on to furniture and walls while navigating, but this should not go on for days and days. This problem with moving will be more pronounced when you can't see, such as at night or when your eyes are closed.

"Unsteady," by the way, can be a description of how you look as you move, or it can describe how you feel. You can feel unsteady without looking unsteady. The unsteadiness in the post-attack phase of Meniere's disease can occur because of the disturbance of your vestibular-movement reflexes and the readjustment your brain is undergoing because of the attack.

After an attack, some people stand and/or walk with their feet further apart than usual. This is part of an unconscious effort to prevent falling. A wider base can create more stability.

Motion intolerance during the aftermath is common. Transient vertigo or nausea can occur during movement that involves your head. The movement can be a turning of your head while your body is still or a turning of your entire body along with your head. These symptoms occur because of the mismatch between what the brain expects and what it gets during head movement.

"For the next three days (after the attack) I was extremely dizzy, couldn't move my head."

—C.D., *On the Level*, Summer 1993

References

_____. U.K. Meniere's Society. *Spin*. Winter 1995.

_____. Vestibular Disorders Association. *On the Level*. Summer 1993, Fall 1996.

Blakley, B.W., and Siegel, M.E. *Feeling Dizzy: Understanding and Treating Vertigo, Dizziness and Other Balance Disorders*. New York: MacMillan, 1995.

Cawthorne, T.E. "Meniere's Disease." *Annals of Otolaryngology—Head and Neck Surgery*, 58:18-37, 1947.

Chalat, N.I. "Who Was Prosper Meniere and Why Am I Still So Dizzy?" *American Journal of Otology*, 1(1):52-56, 1979.

Cleveland, P.J., and Morris, J. "Meniere's Disease: The Inner Ear Out of Balance." *RN*, 54:28-32, 1990.

Conn, H.F. *Conn's Current Therapy*. Philadelphia: W.B. Saunders Company, 1996.

Farber, S.D. "Living with Meniere's Disease: An Occupational Therapist's Perspective." *American Journal of Occupational Therapy*, 43(5): 341-343, 1989.

Yardley, L. *Vertigo and Dizziness*. New York: Routledge, 1994.

Chapter 11

Remission

Otolaryngology textbooks and many journals describe the time between attacks of Meniere's disease as free of symptoms or "normal."

"The most significant feature was the contrast between the prostrating attacks and the intervals—often of weeks or longer—of complete freedom from symptoms of vestibular disturbance."

—T.E. Cawthorne,
Annals of Otolaryngology—Head and Neck Surgery, 1947

"Most patients with Meniere's disease look and feel well between exacerbations."
—S.E. Kinney, et al., *American Journal of Otology*, 1997

Unfortunately, this is not always the case. Only people in the earliest stage of Meniere's disease are free of all symptoms—including tinnitus, hearing loss, and aural pressure—between attacks.

The typical person with Meniere's disease has at least one of the major symptoms all the time and probably has one or more of the adjunctive symptoms also. As described in Chapter 10, "Aftermath," most people experience continuing symptoms in the days immediately following an attack. A few unlucky people have imbalance symptoms all the time. The later stages of Meniere's disease can produce nearly constant symptoms including hearing loss, tinnitus, and balance problems. Even people who are normal (without hearing, tinnitus, aural pressure, or vertigo/balance symptoms) between attacks can have adjunctive problems.

In addition to the main symptoms and adjunctive symptoms such as nausea, cold sweat, and vision disturbances, you may experience symptoms or problems related to living with the constant threat of a disabling attack. Never knowing when and where an attack will occur can cause worry, depression, fear, anger, and frustration, and may cause someone with the disease to lose confidence, self-esteem, and independence and perhaps to stay home most or all of the time.

The symptoms most commonly experienced between attacks by people not in the late stages of Meniere's disease are discussed below.

The symptoms associated with late-stage Meniere's disease can be found in the next chapter.

Hearing

By far the most common symptoms experienced between attacks are related to the cochlea. Low frequency (low-pitched) hearing loss, tinnitus, and aural pressure/pain are present between attacks in a large number of people. However, they are usually not as pronounced as during an attack.

Increased sensitivity to sound (hyperacusis) can also occur. Hyperacusis can be anything from a minor inconvenience to a large problem. Hyperacusis drives some people to wear ear plugs or avoid sound altogether.

Balance

Balance problems are not as common between attacks as the hearing symptoms. Some people have a constant or intermittent problem with unsteadiness after the aftermath. Others report a variety of unpleasant sensations.

"Thankfully I had been in remission from any horrendous attacks all last year and apart from a few "off balance" and "grotty" days, came through unscathed."
—B.E., *Spin*, Summer 1996

"I was plagued with "off" days consisting of muzzy heads, inability to concentrate, and fatigue."
—A.G., *Spin*, Autumn 1995

Vision

Some individuals describe their vision as being "not quite right." Others have found their depth perception to be inaccurate or focusing to be a problem. Blurred vision may also occur. Great care should be taken in situations requiring accurate depth perception such as driving or crossing a road on foot or when focusing is crucial.

"By the middle of August, I was back to where I'd been in February. The floor gave a lurch every now and then and I still had a little trouble focusing, but that was all."
—Chalat, N.I., *American Journal of Otology*, 1979

Glare from house lights, sunlight, and approaching car headlights can be a big problem. Wearing sunglasses outside helps limit the glare of the sun, but you should not wear them to drive at night or when you walk in the dark. Flourescent lights and other things that flicker, such as computer monitor screens, can be annoying or intolerable.

"The flickering screen was the worst. . ."
—E.L., *Spin*, Summer 1996

Thought

Meniere's disease is not a brain disorder or mental illness, but at times it seems to affect thinking. Some people find themselves groping for words; others feel that their short term memory is not quite up to par, and some have problems with writing and spelling.

Emotions

This incurable, chronic illness can cause a variety of negative emotions, such as fear, worry, depression, anger, frustration, and loss of self-reliance and self-esteem. Fear of not being believed, loss of control, loss of social effectiveness, and fears about job loss are common.

"I started to worry that my company would think that I was malingering."
—J.A., *Spin*, Summer 1996

"I lived a haunted life, never feeling safe, always fearing that I would lose control of my world."
—V.G., letter to the author, 1996

". . . am now scared to go out alone as I had an attack outside. . . ."
—A.C., *Spin*, Winter 1995

The fear of falling is a big concern for those over 65 who have Meniere's disease. A fall could result in serious injury such as a fractured hip, could deplete financial resources, and could be life-threatening.

Depression or at least "feeling blue" is common in people with a chronic illness and should not be surprising in people who have had their lives "turned upside down" by the symptoms and the inconsistency of this disease.

"I cannot tell how depressed I get."
—P.C., *Spin*, Winter 1995

Anger is another emotion common to individuals with a chronic illness—anger at having their lives interrupted or changed, anger at the way they are treated or spoken to by other people, anger at not feeling well or at the lack of a definitive treatment.

"The ensuing years found me trying to understand this illness that had changed my life from a confident, understanding, highly involved and level headed person who was able to take life as it came into an angry, unsure, unstable, bad tempered person. . . ."

—C.T., *Spin*, Summer 1995

Frustration is yet another common emotion.

"My husband has this terribly frustrating disease."

—E.L., *Spin*, Summer 1996

The symptoms of Meniere's disease may also cause the loss of self-reliance, self-esteem, and self-confidence.

"I didn't want to go on living. I felt robbed of life, of my potential and God-given talents. I was angry at people with other diseases that seemed more appealing."

—S.T., letter to the author, 1997

"Life after Meniere's is at best described as total modification. A once fiercely independent person becomes very dependent, almost a prisoner at home."

—H. Cohen, *et al.*,
Archives of Otolaryngology—Head and Neck Surgery, 1995.

"My confidence has taken a bashing. . . ."

—J.A., *Spin*, Summer 1996

"I've lost all confidence in getting on buses or going far from home."

—T.H., *Spin*, Winter 1995

All of these can combine to become a terrific burden between the attacks of vertigo, enough to wear down the patience of a saint.

References

_____. U.K. Meniere's Society. *Spin*. Winter 1995, Autumn 1995, Summer 1995, Summer 1996.

Cawthorne, T.E. "Meniere's Disease." *Annals of Otolaryngology—Head and Neck Surgery*, 58:18-37, 1947.

Chalat, N.I. "Who Was Prosper Meniere and Why Am I Still So Dizzy?" *American Journal of Otology*, 1(1):52-56, 1979.

Cohen, H., Ewell, L.R., and Jenkins, H.A. "Disability in Meniere's Disease." *Archives of Otolaryngology—Head and Neck Surgery*, 121:29-33, 1995.

Kinney, S.E., Sandridge, S.A., and Newman, C.W. "Long-Term Effects of Meniere's Disease on Hearing and Quality of Life." *American Journal of Otology,* 18:67-73, 1997.

Merchant, S.N., Rauch, S.D., and Nadol, J.B. "Meniere's Disease." *European Archives of Otorhinolaryngology,* 252:63-75, 1995.

Yardley, L. *Vertigo and Dizziness.* London: Routledge, 1994.

Chapter 12

Late-Stage
Meniere's Disease

W hen Meniere's disease is in its early stages, symptoms many times come and go with the attacks. In its final stages, this may change. Hearing loss stops fluctuating and becomes permanent; tinnitus becomes constant, and the attacks of violent, spontaneous vertigo stop. These final changes in symptoms are sometimes referred to by doctors as "burnout."

Balance

The once violent attacks of vertigo with a symptom-free interval have slowly stopped and in some cases have been replaced by disequilibrium or feelings of unsteadiness.

> "The giddiness I was subject to, instead of coming seldom and violent, now constantly attends me, more or less, though in a more peaceable manner, yet it will not qualify me to live among the young and the healthy."
> —Jonathan Swift, author of *Gulliver's Travels*, as quoted in *American Journal of Otology*, 1979.

Definition: Disequilibrium (sometimes spelled dysequilibrium) is a term used to describe a vague sense of unsteadiness, imbalance, tilting, or bumping into things that can occur in association with vestibular problems. *Dys-* is a prefix meaning difficult or bad. *Dis-* is a prefix meaning negative or absent.

Problems with "balance" can be divided into two categories, symptoms and functions. A balance symptom would refer to feelings you have, such as imbalance, unsteadiness, or of being tilted. A balance function would refer to actions such as staggering, running into things, clumsiness, falling or starting to fall when you close your eyes or turn your head rapidly.

"My head is pretty well, only a sudden turn at any time makes me feel giddy for a moment."

—Martin Luther, as quoted in
American Journal of Otology, 1979.

In those whom the disease progresses to the point of permanently damaging the vestibular parts of the inner ear, balance problems can change from mainly negative symptoms to outward signs of impaired function, particularly in people with Meniere's disease in both ears. Instead of just feeling off-balance and unsteady, you may become visibly off-balance and unsteady. You may misjudge exactly where things are around you and may run into things. Moving around in the dark or on uneven surfaces may be difficult.

There may be subconscious or conscious changes in the way you move around. Some people find themselves touching things while walking, looking down while walking, and standing with their feet wider apart then before. Because the brain is not receiving any information from the affected ear (or the information it is receiving is faulty), the brain begins to use the other senses involved in balance more than before. Vision may be used to verify foot placement, and touch may be used to confirm body position in relation to surrounding objects.

The brain sends out signals so that while you are walking or standing your feet will be further apart to provide a more stable base of support.

About 10 percent of the people with Meniere's disease will experience an episode called Tumarkin's otolithic crisis. You may also hear it referred to as a drop attack, which refers to someone suddenly falling to the ground (an event not confined to people with inner ear problems).

Definition: Someone experiencing **Tumarkin's otolithic crisis** will suddenly fall to the ground without losing consciousness or experiencing vertigo. This person will feel as though he or she has suddenly been pushed, shoved, or knocked to the ground. The crisis is thought to be caused by a sudden problem with the saccule or utricle of the inner ear. (These are the gravity-sensing areas.) Tumarkin's otolithic crisis can occur anytime during Meniere's but is somewhat more common late in the disease.

Because Tumarkin episodes happen without any warning, they can cause serious injury. If you experience one of these episodes, discuss it with your doctor.

Hearing

Late in Meniere's disease, hearing loss is continuous, permanent, and larger than before but will probably not go any further. This loss now extends from the lower pitched sounds up into the higher pitched sounds. The affected ear will probably not be able to understand words spoken at a conversational loudness. Tinnitus will be continuous and probably louder than in the early stages. The aural fullness/pressure may decrease or even disappear altogether.

Vision

During the course of Meniere's disease, the brain has come to depend on vision for some of the information it used to get from the inner ears. Any situation that removes or distorts vision may cause some disequilibrium or loss of balance. Walking with the eyes closed, walking in darkness, trying to look through "steamed" up glasses or goggles, looking through a camera view finder or binoculars or a telescope all have potential for causing problems.

A loss of vestibular function on both sides can cause another visual symptom, oscillopsia (bouncing vision). (See Chapter 5, "Vision.") Without the balance information usually supplied by the ears, the eyes cannot adjust to movement that involves the head. Without this adjustment, everything in your vision will seem to bounce when you move your head. This can even occur when you brush your teeth or chew something crunchy (like an apple or raw carrot). It has even been reported to occur in synchronicity with the heart beat. The bouncing should stop when you stop moving your head, chewing, or brushing your teeth. Your vision will be normal when your head is still unless your heart beat also causes the bouncing.

Keep in mind that not everyone with Meniere's disease experiences these late-stage symptoms. A great many cases of Meniere's disease stop long before reaching this point.

References

Baloh, R.W., Jacobson, K., and Winder, T. "Drop Attacks with Meniere's Syndrome." *Annals of Neurology,* 28(3):384-387, 1990.

Black, F.O., Effron, M.Z., and Burns, D.S. "Diagnosis and Management of Drop Attacks of Vestibular Origin: Tumarkin's Otolithic Crisis." *Otolaryngology-Head and Neck Surgery.* 90(2):256-262, 1982.

Chalat, N.I. "Who Was Prosper Meniere and Why Am I Still So Dizzy?" *American Journal of Otology,* 1(1):52-56, 1979.

Janzen, V.D., and Russell, R.D. "Conservative Management of Tumarkin's Otolithic Crisis." *Journal of Otolaryngology,* 17(7):359-361, 1988.

Merchant, S.N., Rauch, S.D., and Nadol, J.B. "Meniere's Disease." *European Archives of Otorhinolaryngology,* 252:63-75, 1995.

Odkvist, L.M., and Bergenius, J. "Drop Attacks in Meniere's Disease." *Acta Otolaryngologica,* Supplement, 455:82-85, 1988.

Pillsbury, H.C., and Postma, D.S. "Lermoyez' Syndrome and the Otolithic Crisis of Tumarkin. *Otolaryngological Clinics of North America,* 16(1):197-203, 1983.

Pinner, M., and Miller, B.J. *When Doctors Are Patients.* New York: W.W. Norton and Company, Inc., 1952.

Shea, J.J. "Classification of Meniere's Disease." *American Journal of Medicine,* 14(3):224-229, 1993.

Tumarkin, A. "Otolithic Catastrophe: A New Syndrome." *British Medical Journal,* 2:175-177, 1936.

Yardley, L. *Vertigo and Dizziness.* London: Routledge, 1994.

Part III:
Examination and Testing

Doctors use physical examination and testing to assist in the diagnosis of Meniere's disease, to determine a patient's functional status, and to monitor changes related to the disease.

Chapter 13

The Doctor's Examination

I f doctors agree on one thing about Meniere's disease, it is likely to be the importance of getting an accurate and thorough history at the start of the diagnostic process.

What Is a History?

Your medical history includes all the information about your past or present that can help your doctor understand your current health status and assess the problem for which you seek treatment. This means information about the following:

- Your general health
- Your symptoms, both major and minor
- What you feel during an attack
- What you were doing when the symptoms first appeared
- Whether you were doing anything such as scuba diving, sky diving, or flying in an unpressurized airplane that might have caused the symptoms
- When the symptoms occur
- If the symptoms are spontaneous or if some specific activity or circumstance brings them on
- How long they stay
- How strong they are
- How often they come
- How many times you have had them
- If they include nausea or vomiting
- If there is a warning
- If anything makes the symptoms better
- If anything makes them worse
- If you have ever had anything like them
- If you have any relatives with similar symptoms
- If you have had ear infections or ear problems
- If you have ever had allergies or hay fever

- If you have ever had migraines
- Any diseases, problems, accidents, or injuries you have had
- What drugs you are taking or have taken in the not too distant past
- Any treatments you may be undergoing and the purpose for the treatments
- Any special diet you are on and why
- The general health of your closest relatives

Why Is a Medical History So Important?

Most vestibular disorders cannot be distinguished from one another solely on the basis of testing. In other words, most of the relevant tests show only that abnormalities do or do not exist, not where in your vestibular system an abnormality lies or the exact nature of the problem. Without complete knowledge of the symptoms and the rest of your story, the test results may not lead to an accurate diagnosis.

The Examination

Generally your doctor first wants to know whether your symptoms result from a problem that can cause great harm in the immediate future. Luckily, most causes of dizziness, including Meniere's disease, will not directly cause loss of limb or life. In fact, all inner ear causes of vertigo are considered "benign." In this context, benign means they won't kill you even though they may disrupt your life.

In general, someone experiencing vertigo but no symptoms of a problem in the cochlea will undergo the most extensive examinations by one or more specialists. Their examinations might include a look at other systems such as the cardiovascular system and the nervous system (including the brain).

An otolaryngologist's examination of someone with dizziness usually focuses on the following:
- Hearing
- Ear
- Nose/sinuses and throat
- Brain and nervous system
- Eye movement
- Balance and movement

Hearing

Your hearing may be checked by an audiologist before you see the doctor, as described in Chapter 15, "Hearing Tests," or your oto-laryngologist might also have you listen to a tuning fork(s) placed behind your ears or on your forehead. You might be asked to compare sounds or say when a sound disappears.

Ear

The external ear canal can be examined directly for obstruction by things such as wax, infection, or foreign bodies. The tympanic membrane (ear drum) can be checked for holes (perforations), signs of fluid or infection in the middle ear, and for a middle ear growth called a cholesteatoma.

Nose, Sinuses, and Throat

The nose, sinuses, and throat are checked for inflammation, swelling, infection, or any other abnormality.

Brain and Nervous System

Your doctor will check the function and condition of your brain indirectly by checking a number of things such as how well you can answer questions, how your eyes move, what your eye pupils look like and how they react to light, and how you move muscles around your face. The doctor may also check your muscle strength and coordination, and your reflexes, and might also test your senses of smell, taste, touch, and vision.

Balance and Movement

For a quick look at your balance function, your doctor will have you stand with your feet side by side and eyes closed or with one foot in front of the other and might also have you "march in place," stand on one foot, or stand on your toes. The doctor may also push you a bit while you are standing. He or she will have you walk in your normal way, may ask you to walk by placing one foot in front of the other or heel to toe, and may have you walk backwards. Possibly, you may be asked to stand on a cushion or walk on something soft.

A pressure test may be done. The air pressure in your external auditory canal is changed while your eyes are observed for any abnormal movement. You may also be asked if you feel anything different during this pressure change.

Eye Movement

Your doctor will observe your eyes for nystagmus while your head is still, when you are moving your head, when you are following the doctor's finger with your eyes, and possibly when your doctor is moving your head or when you are in different positions. He or she may check your vision with a standard wall chart while you stand still or possibly while you move your head. You might be asked to put on a pair of glasses or goggles (Frenzel lenses). (See Figure 13-1.) These magnify your eyes for the examiner and force you to look through lenses you cannot focus with. This prevents you from fixing your vision on something, which would make it difficult for the doctor to see eye movement abnormalities that might be present.

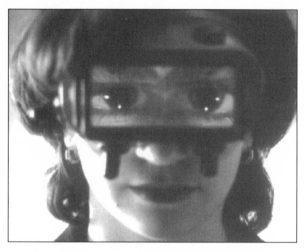

Figure 13-1:
Frenzel lenses
(Photo courtesy of ICS Medical Corporation, Schaumburg, Illinois.)

Feeling Dizzy: Understanding and Treating Vertigo, Dizziness and Other Balance Disorders by Brian W. Blakeley, M.D., and Mary-Ellen Siegel, M.S.W. (MacMillan, 1995), includes an excellent in-depth description of the kind of examination a newly dizzy person may undergo.

Chapter 14

Testing—
Introduction

In addition to obtaining a history and doing an examination (covered in Chapter 13, "The Doctor's Examination"), many doctors use tests to help make the diagnosis of Meniere's disease, to determine a patient's functional status, and to monitor changes.

However, no standard battery of tests exists to diagnose Meniere's disease. Each doctor usually has his or her own selection of tests for ruling out other conditions and then making the diagnosis. The way these tests are conducted is also not standardized. (This can become a bit of a problem if you switch doctors.)

Difficulty With Testing

Why Is the Inner Ear Difficult to Study and Test?

Tiny and embedded within the densest bone of the body, the interior of the inner ear can't be seen or visualized with currently available technology (ultrasound, X-Ray, CT scan, MRI). The inner ear also cannot be entered with any instrument without risking total loss of hearing and vestibular function. In addition, although signals from the cochlea to the brain can be recorded and evaluated, signals from the vestibular apparatus to the brain cannot.

Why Is It Difficult to Test for Meniere's Disease?

• The cause is unknown.
• No other mammals are known to naturally develop Meniere's disease; therefore no satisfactory animal is available to study. (Endolymphatic hydrops can be artificially created in research ani-

mals, but this does not provide entirely the same data that natural-ly occurring hydrops could provide.)

- The vestibular apparatus has multiple parts, and its function is complicated because it constantly senses gravity and movement in a number of directions simultaneously. It also sends about 100 signals per second to the brain at all times.
- Hearing tests can assess hearing, but no tests exist to verify the presence of tinnitus, aural pressure, or most of the other symptoms accompanying Meniere's disease. For this, your doctor must depend totally on what you say.
- Vestibular tests don't directly measure the work of the vestibular apparatus. Instead they measure the function of two vestibular reflexes, the vestibulo-ocular reflex and the vestibulo-spinal reflex.
- Hearing tests are good but test only the hearing function of the middle ear, cochlea, cochlear branch of the acoustic nerve, and the hearing pathways of the brainstem. To make a diagnosis of Meniere's disease with the aid of hearing tests, your doctor must assume that the excess endolymph thought to be causing your hearing problem is also affecting your vestibular areas.

Your Testing

If your doctor wants you to undergo a battery of tests, you might want to ask the following questions:

- What do these tests look at or for?
- Are any risks or dangers involved?
- If so, what alternative tests exist?

If you have questions about your testing, try to discuss them with your doctor or your doctor's staff. (The audiologist may be able to answer your questions.) They are the only ones who can tell you why they did or did not request a certain test and what the results mean in your particular case. If for some reason you feel under-tested and belong to an HMO or other managed care arrangement, ask your doctor if any tests have been left out solely at the request of the insurance company or to save money. Don't assume you would be told this if it was a factor.

Note about insurance: If you are with an HMO (health maintenance organization), do not go for a test unless you have the proper referral. If you are with a PPO (preferred provider organization), make sure the doctor or testing place is on the "approved" list. Sometimes a chat beforehand with the insurance billing clerk at your doctor's office or the testing center can alert you to potential insurance problems.

Why Hasn't My Doctor Done All the Tests I Hear Other People Have Had?

Your doctor may have many reasons for ordering or not ordering a particular test. The test may be unnecessary given your symptoms and circumstances; your doctor may feel the test is not useful; it may be unavailable in your geographic location; it might cost more money than an insurance company wants to spend (particularly in the case of HMOs and other "managed care" kinds of insurance); a large hearing loss can make some tests impossible to do; your insurance carrier may consider a test or tests experimental, inappropriate, redundant, or "unnecessary," and/or your doctor might not know about the test or understand it fully enough to use it.

Basic Testing Concepts

Test Categories

The testing can be divided into three categories: tests of hearing, tests of vestibular function, and miscellaneous tests. Hearing is measured "directly," and balance function is mostly measured "indirectly." All the hearing tests involve sound in some way. The tests of vestibular function may be referred to as balance tests, but the majority actually observe or measure eye movement. Because of the vestibular-ocular reflex, the eyes are something of a window on the inner ear.

Test Goals

• To determine the side or sides involved
• To decide if the problem is in the ear or elsewhere
• To rule out the presence of a tumor

Testing and Drugs

It is important to follow your doctor's instructions about what drugs can be taken or not taken before and during testing and for how long. When health professionals refer to "medications" or "drugs" in this context, they mean prescription drugs and non-prescription drugs like aspirin and street drugs such as cocaine.

Your doctor will not want you to take medications that can interfere with testing, but he or she also will **not** want you to stop taking any medications, such as insulin, heart drugs, blood pressure medications, that are essential for treating other conditions. If in addition to your suspected inner ear problems you have conditions that require medication on a regular schedule or as needed, discuss them with your doctor.

Some drugs can cover up abnormalities that must be observed or measured during testing, and other drugs can create abnormalities. The following table lists some common drugs known to interfere with accurate testing.

Table 14-1: Drugs That May Impede Testing

Dilantin (phenytoin)	marijuana
Tegretol (carbamazepine)	lithium
barbiturates	Antivert (meclizine)
methadone	Elavil
nicotine gum	imipramine
tobacco	Benadryl (dimenhydrinate)
Valium (diazepam)	quinine*
Xanax (alprazolam)	amitriptyline
alcohol	tranquilizers in general
Librium (chlordiazepoxide)	sedatives in general
Ativan (lorazepam)	aspirin ^

* A list of substances containing quinine can be found on page 248.
^ A list of substances containing aspirin can be found on page 247.

Testing and Allergies

Many of the tests use "sticky patches," electrodes that are stuck to the body, usually on the face and/or head. These usually contain water, glycerol, and polyacrylic acid (containing sodium sulfonate groups). If you are allergic to any of these, notify your doctor's office and the testing center.

Testing and "Conscious Manipulation"

Meniere's disease is a disease of symptoms. Symptoms are entirely subjective; only the person experiencing them knows what they are like, when they are present, and what effect they have. Someone with Meniere's disease does not have a certain look and usually does not have any outward signs of a "balance" problem. (This is the general case between attacks in early Meniere's disease but is not the case during attacks.)

Sometimes people undergoing examination and testing may feel that their symptoms and the problems created by them have been minimized or ignored by the health care professionals they have encountered. In an attempt to make their symptoms and difficulties visible during testing or examination, they may choose not to walk or stand in place to the best of their ability, or they may allow themselves to fall when they could prevent it.

Exaggeration of disability can lead to the wrong diagnosis and treatment or cause doubt in the examiner's mind about whether or not you have a physical problem. It's in your best interest during an examination or testing procedure to carry on to the best of your ability. Don't yield to the temptation to "show them how you feel."

Disclaimer

As you read chapters on testing, keep in mind that VEDA and this author do not mean to endorse or disavow the tests described here. We are not suggesting that all these tests be performed to diagnose Meniere's disease or to rule out (exclude) other conditions. We are describing the examination and tests to help explain what they measure, what they are like, and for what reasons (other than diagnosis) they might be used. VEDA and the author are not suggesting the use of one or another of the tests in a particular situation.

Chapter 15

Hearing Tests

The tests most commonly performed to diagnose Meniere's disease are measurements of hearing, as follows:

- "ordinary" hearing test (also called an audiogram or "audio")

- glycerol test

- electrocochleography (ECoG)

These not only check the amount of hearing, they are also important in determining the location of the loss — either the middle ear or the complex consisting of the cochlea, acoustic nerve, and brain. These tests are important because they can help determine not only if a problem exists in the cochlea but which ear is the "problem" ear.

What Do These Tests Reveal About Your Dizziness?

The cochlea and vestibular apparatus are connected to each other and share the same two inner ear fluids. A test suggesting increased endolymph in the cochlea also suggests increased endolymph in the vestibular areas.

"Ordinary" Hearing Test

Since fluctuating sensorineural hearing loss (in the low frequencies in early Meniere's) is one of the three major symptoms of Meniere's disease and the only one that can be measured easily and accurately, the test for this loss is performed most often.

Preparation for the Test

The hearing test requires no preparation or instructions beforehand. Just show up on time and follow any instructions given by the audiologist. Since you must consciously participate in the test, go as well-rested and as relaxed as you can.

What Is It Like?

First, middle ear function is checked. An ear plug is inserted into the external auditory canal, and the air pressure is both increased and decreased automatically by computer to measure the ability of the tympanic membrane to move. This is done one ear at a time and should be painless. Figure 15-1 shows the results of such a test, a tympanogram.

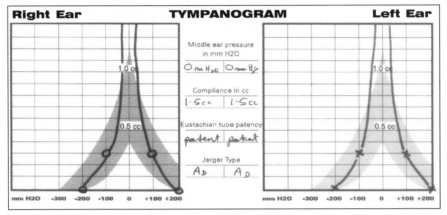

Figure 15-1: Tympanogram. The shaded area shaped like a teepee is the normal range. (Courtesy of Dr. A. K. Chaudri and Dr. S. A. Chaudri, Bombay, India.)

The hearing test is done in a sound-proof booth using headphones to assure that the only things you can hear are the audiologist and the test sounds. Both sounds and speech are used. A series of tones at several pitches (also called frequencies) are presented to each ear. You are asked to respond when you hear the tone by raising your hand or pressing a button, and the audiologist determines at what loudness (also called decibel level) you heard it. Sometimes, in addition to the pure tones, a sound similar to radio static, called masking, is used.

Another part of the hearing test determines how well you recognize spoken words (speech discrimination) and at what decibel level (speech reception threshold) you can understand them. The audiologist will ask you to repeat each word he or she says or perhaps will play a tape with words to repeat. Your speech discrimination will be recorded as the percentage of single syllable words that you successfully repeat. Your speech reception threshold will be the loudness or decibel level at which you can understand half of the equally weighted two-syllable words well enough to repeat them successfully. ("Baseball" is an example of a two-syllable equal-weight word.)

You may also be tested for recruitment at this time. Recruitment is the perception of an abnormally rapid growth of loudness when sound intensity is increased. In other words, when a sound's loudness increases, an ear with recruitment senses this increase more rapidly than does a normal ear. This effect is thought to be common in Meniere's disease.

What Do These Hearing Tests Show?

The tests show whether or not your middle ear function is normal. It will be normal if your tympanic membrane and eustachian tube are working properly and your middle ear cavity does not contain fluid.

If a hearing loss is present, the tests will show at what frequency it occurs, at what decibel level, and whether it involves the middle ear or the cochlea/nerve/brain.

The tests will also reveal speech discrimination ability; that is, how well speech is understood, and whether the speech discrimination score is consistent with the level of hearing. (Speech discrimination in Meniere's disease usually decreases proportionately to hearing loss.) A hearing loss in the lower frequencies that fluctuates from visit to visit would be consistent with the hearing loss of early stage Meniere's disease. In the later stages, a hearing loss can also be found in the upper frequencies and might not fluctuate.

Other Uses

Hearing tests may also be done at regular intervals to check on the degree of hearing fluctuation and hearing loss. This testing can also be used to determine if a hearing aid would be beneficial.

After the Test

The audiologist or doctor will probably show you the results of the test. These results are plotted on a graph with the pitch or frequency along one axis and the decibel level or loudness along another. The best possible theoretical result would be to hear each frequency (pitch) at the 0 decibel level. Figure 15-2 shows a sample of a right ear audiogram.

Figure 15-3 depicts the decibel and frequency levels of normal speech.

A low frequency loss would lie between 250 hz and 750 hz. A middle frequency loss would occur between 1,000 hz and 3,000 hz. A high frequency loss would lie between 4,000 hz and 8,000 hz. The ranges from 750 to 1,000 hz and from 3,000 to 4,000 hz are not tested. Figure 15-4 illustrates how scores in the various areas of the graph are classified.

The decibel levels of a selection of common sounds are listed in Table 15-1, page 110. Also see Chapter 34, "Preservation, Protection" for related information, including OSHA guidelines for noise exposure.

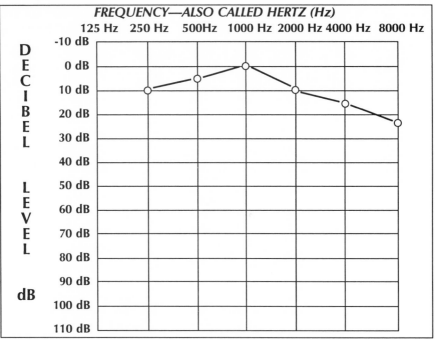

Figure 15-2: Audiogram for a right ear, represented by a series of Os. A left ear would be represented by Xs.

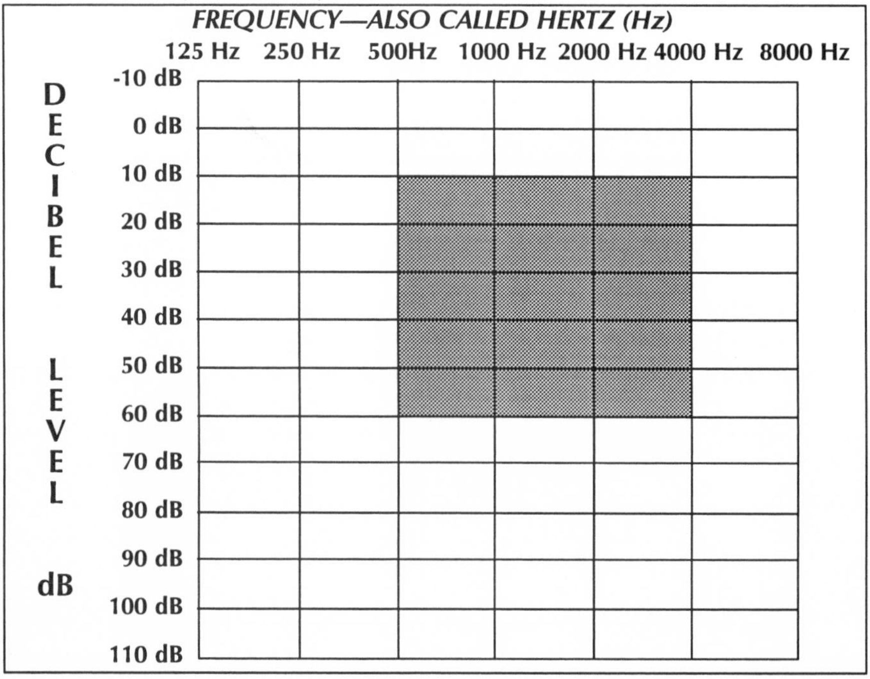

Figure 15-3: Frequencies and decibel levels of **human speech** (shaded box).

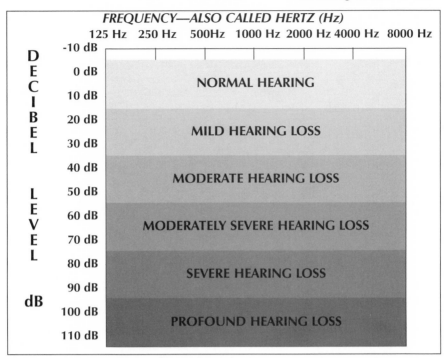

Figure 15-4: Hearing loss classifications.

Glycerol Test

This is the "ordinary" hearing test with a twist. A chemical is used in an attempt to "dehydrate" the inner ear. The glycerol test is also sometimes called a dehydration test or glycerol dehydration test.

Preparation for the Test

The staff of the doctor's office or testing place should provide complete instructions about any preparation for this test, when to arrive, and how much time to allow for the testing. Generally speaking, you will be asked to abstain from food and drink for several hours before the test so that the glycerol can work without any interference. Sometimes this test is done in coordination with an ECoG, explained below.

What Is It Like?

Your hearing is tested, and then you are asked to drink a chilled liquid, usually glycerol, that most people would describe as having an unpleasant, sweet taste. The hearing is tested again at

Table 15-1: Decibel Levels of Common Sounds		
140	nearby thunder	air raid siren
130	machine-gun fire at close range	jackhammer
120	jet plane 200 feet away air hammer	firecracker
110	chain saw jet flying 1,000 feet overhead ambulance siren	snowmobile rock music
100	power mower	
90	food blender	
80	clothes washer garbage disposal doorbell	dishwasher alarm clock
70	television vacuum cleaner	car at 65 mph from 25 feet
60	conversation	
50	classroom	loud rain
40	singing birds	
30	whisper	
20	rustling leaves	
10	ordinary breathing (barely audible)	

intervals spaced over a total of about three hours to see if the hearing level changes.

How Does It Work?

The idea is that the glycerol (an osmotic agent) will chemically "pull" some of the excess endolymph out of the cochlea, thus allowing the hearing to improve if the cochlear hearing loss is still reversible. This movement of fluid usually only occurs in early Meniere's disease, not with late-stage disease.

What Does It Show?

Improved hearing during the test is thought to indicate that the inner ear is being affected by the excess endolymph of Meniere's disease. However, unchanged hearing during the test does not rule out Meniere's disease.

Other Uses

In the past, this test has been used to assess for the appropriateness of endolymphatic shunt or valve surgery of the inner ear.

After the Test

You should experience no long-term ill effects from this test. However, it is not uncommon to experience nausea, diarrhea, lightheadedness, and fatigue in the immediate period after the test. Plan to have someone drive you home from the test, or allow enough time to recover before driving.

ECoG

This is a different, more sophisticated type of hearing test. ECoG is an abbreviation for electrocochleography, also called ECochG or cochlear evoked potentials.

Preparation for the Test

Staff at the doctor's office or testing place should provide information about any preparation necessary such as not eating or drinking for a time, when to arrive, and how much time to allow for testing. You may be asked to abstain from diuretics ("water" pills) for a time before the test. The test can also be done in conjunction with a glycerol test. (See above.)

What Is It Like?

In the main variation of this test, called the "extratympanic EcoG," a wire called an electrode is placed in the external ear canal or on the ear drum. In some testing places, the wire electrode is connected to a needle which is inserted through the ear drum into the middle ear; this variation of the test is called "transtympanic EcoG." Sticky patches connected to wires (electrodes) are placed on a few areas around your head, usually on your face and ear lobes. You will be asked to rest comfortably while listening to a series of click-like sounds and possibly a sound like the ringing of a wind-up alarm clock. You are not to respond in any way, just relax. (The pressure test done by some doctors in conjunction with EcoG is an exception. It involves holding the breath and bearing down as instructed.)

In depth (transtympanic ECoG): The transtympanic ECoG is also referred to as a TT ECoG. After the tympanic membrane has been sprayed with anesthetic, a needle connected to an electrode is passed through it and the tip of the needle is positioned near the cochlea. This kind of ECoG provides the most accurate waveform but is more invasive than the extratympanic variety. Theoretical risks of the TT ECoG include infection and persistent ear drum perforation (hole). Check with your doctor or the staff of the testing center for complete details. When discussing risks, ask not only "What are they?" but "How frequently do they occur?"

When an ECoG is performed with glycerol, at least two tests will be done, one before the glycerol and another afterwards.

How Does It Work?

ECoG is a computerized test measuring the way a specific sound moves electrically through the cochlea and the ear end of the vestibulo-cochlear nerve (on the beginning of its trip to the brain). An insert earphone in the ear canal introduces specific, measured sound into the ear. The sticky patches on the head and the electrode in the ear canal sense the electrical changes in the cochlea and beginning of the acoustic nerve and send this information to the computer, which generates a waveform (graph).

In depth (waveform): To describe the results of an ECoG as negative or positive is an oversimplification. What the audiologist actually sees is referred to as a "waveform". Waveforms are graphic representations of the electrical activity created by sound in the cochlea and cochlear branch of the acoustic nerve. They also represent a ratio between two things called the AP and the SP. Your ECoG waveform will be measured to see if it's like the waveform thought to be typical of Meniere's disease.

What Does It Show?

If hydrops is present, it can cause the waveform to have a characteristic shape. Hydrops is thought to interfere with sound transmission within the cochlea and to distort electrical potentials within the cochlea.

Doctors who routinely request the test feel that when it is positive, changes related to Meniere's disease are present in the cochlea, and when the test is negative, Meniere's disease could still be present.

Other Uses

This test has been performed during inner ear surgery to evaluate waveform changes during the operation.

Chapter 16

Indirect Vestibular Function Tests

No available tests can "see" inside the vestibular apparatus or directly measure the balance information going to the brain via the vestibulo-cochlear nerve. The tests can't directly determine if the vestibular apparatus is working normally. However, tests can investigate vestibular function indirectly by looking at two reflexes that depend on vestibular information. These reflexes are called the vestibulo-ocular reflex (VOR) and the vestibulo-spinal reflex (VSR).

Although tests can point toward a vestibular problem, they may not be able to determine which problem or sometimes tell which ear is at fault. If vertigo is the only symptom, determining which ear is at fault is a big problem. With Meniere's disease, it's the other symptoms—hearing loss, tinnitus, and aural pressure—that help identify the problem ear.

The available tests look at the function of the VOR and that of the VSR and provide indirect methods of checking on vestibular function. These indirect tests include ENG, rotational tests, and computerized dynamic posturography.

Note: Unlike hearing tests, these tests do not always determine which side has the problem.

General Preparation for These Tests

Complete instructions should be provided by the staff of the doctor's office or the testing center about any preparation necessary such as not eating or drinking for a time, when to show up, and how much time to allow for testing. Test instructions may require that you come for the test(s) with an empty stomach.

In general, anti-vertigo drugs and any other drugs that could affect the test results are stopped 24 to 48 hours before the test. Drugs such as meclizine (Antivert), Dramamine, Phenergan, Compazine, and pain killers can interfere with the test. If you have any questions about drugs, call your doctor's office or the test facility staff for clarification.

Most of these tests include placing sticky patches connected to wires (electrodes) on areas (cleaned just prior to attachment) around your face.

For these tests, you should wear comfortable clothing. If you are a woman, you might be more comfortable if you don't wear a dress or skirt, and you should definitely wear slacks or shorts if your tests include posturography. A sweat-suit or warm-up suit might be most comfortable.

If you have a neck or back problem, inform your doctor and the staff at the testing place before going for the testing.

If you have a false eye, need glasses to see beyond the tip of your nose, use contact lenses, or have a visual problem called strabismus, tell the audiologist before the start of the test.

ENG (Electronystagmography)

"ENG" is a label commonly used improperly in referring to a group or battery of eye movement tests that look for signs of vestibular dysfunction or neurological problems. This common use is inaccurate because not all ENG tests involve nystagmus, and the health professionals who conduct these tests are often looking at eye movements other than nystagmus. However, because these tests are so commonly referred to as "an ENG," we will do so to avoid confusion.

Although called electronystagmography, the ENG can measure more than just nystagmus (abnormal eye jerking). It can also record other eye movements having nothing to do with vestibular function. ENG tests are probably the most common of the tests administered to people with dizziness, vertigo, and/or balance disorders, but neither the test battery nor the testing method are standardized.

Special note: If you are scheduled to have an ENG test and by chance have an attack before the test, try to get to the test anyway. Recording eye movement during an actual attack will provide more information to your doctor than any of the tests described in this chapter.

Insurance/billing note: If you receive itemized medical bills for this battery of tests, you will probably find a list of different tests. The initials "ENG" most likely will not appear on the bills.

An ENG can include the following tests:
- visual tracking (can also be called visual-ocular control, ocular dysmetria testing)
- optokinetic nystagmus
- optokinetic after-nystagmus

- saccades testing
- smooth pursuit
- spontaneous nystagmus
- gaze
- positional
- positioning (Hallpike)
- fistula or pressure testing
- head shaking
- caloric (may also be called bithermal caloric, monothermal caloric)

Special Instruction

Blinking interferes with interpretation of the test. Try hard not to blink during the test.

What Is It Like?

The test and its preparation generally require at least 60 minutes. First, areas around your eyes will be cleaned and sticky-patch electrodes applied so that your eye movements can be electrically monitored during the test. See Figure 16-1 for an example.

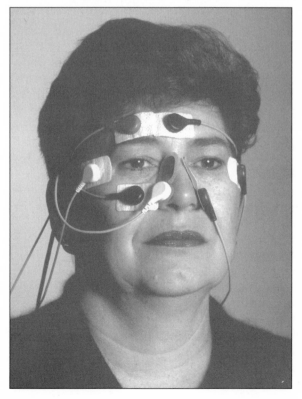

Figure 16-1: Sticky-patch electrodes. A woman prepared for ENG testing. (Courtesy of Micromedical Technologies, Chatham, Illinois.

During this testing, the person in charge will give you a great many instructions, such as to follow this or that with your eyes, stare at this or that, stare at something moving, stare at something stationary, follow a target with your eyes, move your eyes from here to there, close your eyes, open your eyes, turn your head, roll on your side, or count backwards from 100 by threes.

You will be asked to move into different positions from sitting up to lying down on one side or another or turning your head to one side or another. Most of these position changes are slow except for the "Hallpike" or positioning test. In this test, your doctor or other professional will help you rapidly change from sitting to lying with your head to one side and lower than your body (called the head-hanging position). After a short time, you will be returned rapidly to a sitting position. After a rest, you will repeat the procedure on the opposite side.

During the fistula or pressure test, an ear plug will be placed in the external auditory canal of one ear, through which positive and negative pressure will be introduced while your eye movement is measured. Your doctor will test one ear at a time.

The caloric test is generally done last. The majority of people having an ENG find this test to be the most uncomfortable and memorable because it can cause temporary vertigo accompanied by nausea.

The most commonly administered caloric test has four parts and is called the bithermal alternating caloric. The temperature in the external auditory canal of each ear is temporarily changed by a few degrees a total of four times (first ear warm, second ear warm, first ear cool, second ear cool). Your doctor or other professional will probably slide a catheter into your ear canal to deliver air or water to induce the temperature change. The reaction of the eyes (nystagmus) to this change will be measured while you perform a mental task such as counting backwards from 100 by subtracting threes or naming things starting with a certain letter.

Note: Some physicians change the temperature in both ears simultaneously instead of the more standard alternation method, and others change the temperature only once rather than twice.

The temperature change causes a spinning sensation for a short time. The most intense spinning occurs about 60 seconds into the test. The strength of the spinning depends upon the amount of vestibular function present. A normal ear will produce the greatest spinning response. The absence of spinning during this part of the test indicates that vestibular function is absent on the side being tested. If this occurs, the audiologist may retry the test with ice water.

At some point after the entire temperature change has occurred, you will be asked to fix your vision on something straight ahead, such as a red light or a dot on the ceiling. This visual fixation will stop the nystagmus and spinning caused by the temperature change. This procedure will be repeated for each of the four parts of the test.

A further word about the caloric test. It is normal and expected for vertigo to occur when the warm and cool water or air are introduced one at a time into the ear canal. If vertigo does not occur, the test is considered abnormal. This vertigo occurs simultaneously with the nystagmus, (abnormal jerking eye movement) recorded during the test. Fixing your vision on a light or dot on the ceiling when instructed to will usually stop the more intense vertigo by stopping the nystagmus. (This is a tactic used by many people to lessen their vertigo during an attack of Meniere's disease) Some people with Meniere's disease find the spinning caused by the caloric test to be similar or identical to the spinning they experience during attacks, while others feel their attack spinning is not as strong.

Note: Some testing centers use infra-red goggles instead of sticky patch electrodes. When you are tested with goggles, your eyes are kept open all of the time. The goggles look a bit like ski goggles and are a bit more comfortable than electrodes.

Unlike the electrode method, the goggle method doesn't rely on recording the electricity generated by eye movement. Instead this computerized test "sees" the eyes during the test and can pick up any movement, including rotary and vertical, not just horizontal.

What Do These Tests Show?

None of the tests show anything that can be interpreted specifically as Meniere's disease unless an actual attack occurs during the test. In the early stages of Meniere's disease, all the tests should be normal; decreased function will only be apparent during the later stages. A reduced response to the caloric test only tells your doctor that there is a problem either with the horizontal canal of the inner ear, the acoustic nerve, or the brain on a certain side. It cannot indicate that the cause of the reduced response is located solely within the inner ear.

To try to identify the problem ear in people whose only symptom is vertigo, doctors can perform the pressure and caloric tests. If nystagmus or increased symptoms occur when the pressure or temperature in just one ear canal is changed, the problem side may be determined.

In some cases, eye movement tests can point toward a brain problem rather than an inner ear problem or an inner ear problem rather than a brain problem. Certain types of nystagmus come from specific areas of the brain; their presence will point to a problem in those areas. Sometimes the ENG does not reveal any problems but, unfortunately, this does not rule out the possibility of Meniere's disease. The caloric test can also reveal eye abnormalities caused by brain problems.

In depth (nystagmus): Nystagmus is an abnormal jerking of the eyes that can be horizontal (back and forth), vertical (up and down), or rotatory (circular). It has two parts or phases, a slow and a fast. The slow phase is created by the vestibular system and the fast phase by the brain. The eyes slowly move toward one vestibular apparatus and the brain snaps the eyes back to center once their drifting away is noticed.

The amount and direction of the nystagmus is used to help determine if a problem is in the brain or in the inner ear and which ear is the "problem" ear. Figure 16-2 is a graphic representation of horizontal nystagmus.

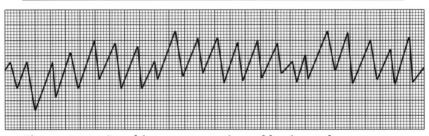

Figure 16-2: Graphic representation of horizontal nystagmus.
(Courtesy of ICS Medical Corporation, Schaumburg, Illinois.)

What Should This Test Show If I Have Meniere's Disease?

If you are not having an attack and don't have permanent vestibular damage, your test results will be probably be normal. If you have permanent vestibular damage, your doctor will probably be able to identify the side of the damage and give an estimate of the degree of damage. If you are lucky enough to be tested during an attack, your nystagmus will be recorded and compared with the type thought to occur during an attack of Meniere's disease. (That nystagmus goes through a series of movements in three directions, toward the "bad" ear, away from the bad ear, and back toward the bad ear).

Other Uses

Like the hearing test, the ENG test battery may be used to periodically monitor your condition after a diagnosis has been made.

After the Test

This test should not cause an attack of Meniere's disease (vertigo with hearing loss and increased tinnitus, or aural pressure). It can cause nausea, fatigue, and a temporary off-balance sensation. Plan to have someone drive you home from the test, or allow enough time to recover before driving.

Rotary Chair

Rotational or turning tests are often used in the diagnosis of Meniere's disease. They are designed to look at the vestibulo-ocular reflex. The rotational tests include both passive and active tests. During a passive test, you will be moved by a machine or by another person. During an active test, you will do the moving yourself.

One of these tests, the rotary chair test, may also be called SHAT or SHA for "sinusoidal harmonic acceleration test." This is a computerized, passive, objective test of the horizontal vestibulo-ocular reflex (VOR). The SHAT may also be referred to as total body rotational testing.

One property of the VOR is that when vision is absent (in darkness or with the eyes closed), turning the head in one direction results in movement of the eyes at exactly the same time and rate of speed in the opposite direction. The rotary chair test is designed to examine this property.

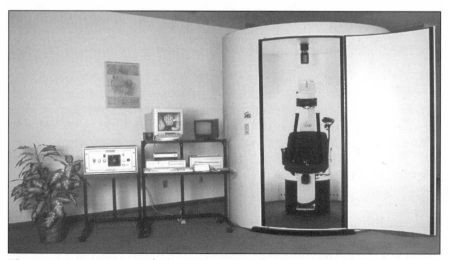

Figure 16-3: Rotary chair. (Courtesy of Micromedical Technologies, Chatham, Illinois.)

What Is It Like?

The test is done in a small room while you sit in a motor-driven computerized chair with your head flexed forward a bit and the lights turned off. Before beginning the test, the person in charge of the test will clean areas of your face, apply electrodes to the clean areas, and put headphones on your head to enable constant contact with the audiologist outside the room. The test and its preparation generally require 40 to 45 minutes.

The test itself has two general parts, chair movement and visual testing. The chair usually moves slowly back and forth through 180 degrees, not around in a full circle. During chair movement, you will not be asked to participate in any way other than to speak with the audiologist at times. (In a few testing centers, the chair movement is faster.) During the visual gaze section, you will be asked to find and follow a little red light with your eyes. Some testing places also add another part, the optokinetic drum test, with the room lights on.

What Does It Show?

The rotary chair test shows how well the central nervous system is processing vestibular information and how well the brain integrates visual/vestibular information. This test shows how the VOR is working and how well you can fix your vision on something. Your doctor wants to know if your eyes move at the same speed as the movement of the chair and how long it takes for your eyes to move once the chair moves.

The test can, at times, show the presence of a vestibular problem but does not usually help identify which ear has the problem because both sides are stimulated simultaneously. No rotary chair result by itself specifically identifies Meniere's disease.

After the Test

This test should not have any long-term effect on you or your vestibular symptoms. If your symptoms are aggravated by movement, plan to have someone drive you home from the test, or allow enough time to stay at the testing center until your symptoms resolve.

Comparison

The rotary chair test requires a computerized moving chair in its own special little room. The test is done at a slower speed than the other two rotational tests (the HSVOR and head-only auto-rotational testing, described below). During the test, your head and body move as a unit; the head does not rotate alone, and it is passive rather than active. The rotary chair test is more standardized from clinic to clinic than the ENG battery.

Many people find the rotary chair test easier and more comfortable than caloric testing.

Other Uses

The SHAT can be used to assess how the brain is "compensating" for a permanent loss of vestibular function and can be used over time to look at this phenomenon. (See Chapter 31, "Compensation.") It is also used, sometimes, over time to assess how someone is doing and is a good test for assessing people with bilateral losses.

Head-Shaking Test (HSVOR)

Another rotational test, the head-shaking test is also called the head-shaking vestibulo-ocular reflex test or HSVOR. It is usually a non-computerized, passive test. (Someone will move your head for you.)

What Is It Like?

The HSVOR is done while you sit, usually wearing Frenzel lenses. The doctor or audiologist moves your head back and forth with his or her hands and observes your eyes for nystagmus.

What Does It Show?

This test produces nystagmus, the speed and direction of which are observed and sometimes recorded. An abnormal test can suggest a problem with the vestibulo-ocular reflex, either in the inner ear, the vestibular nerve, or the brain. No specific HSVOR result establishes the presence of Meniere's disease.

After the Test

Although it can cause temporary fatigue and a feeling of imbalance, this test should not have any long-term effect on you or your symptoms. If your symptoms are aggravated by movement, plan to have someone drive you home from the test, or stay at the testing center until your symptoms resolve.

Auto-Rotational Testing

A third type of rotational test, the auto-rotational test, is a computerized test objectively measuring your ability to keep your eyes focused on a stationary target during active head movement, both back and forth and up and down. The test is also referred to as a head-on-body rotation test, a head-only auto-rotational test, an active head rotation test, a vestibular auto-rotation test (VAT), or a vestibulo-ocular reflex testing equipment (VORTEQ) test. It can test the VOR both horizontally and vertically.

What Is It Like?

Electrodes are placed on your face to measure eye movement, and a device resembling a head band is placed around your head to measure the speed of any head movement. (See Figure 16-4.) While in a sitting position, you are asked to move your head back and forth in time with a sound for no longer than 18 seconds while looking at a visual target (usually a dot) close by. This visual target may appear to jump during the test, but it actually remains stationary. The procedure is repeated twice more at different speeds and then, after a short pause, you will be asked to repeat the performance substituting up-and-down movements for back-and-forth movements. This test requires about 20 minutes including preparation time.

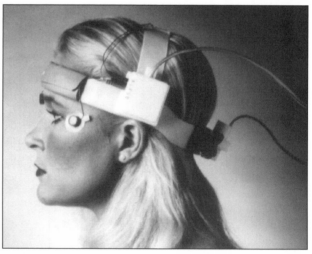

Figure 16-4: Vestibular auto-rotation test (VAT). (Courtesy of Western Systems Research, Pasadena California.)

What Does It Show?

This test shows how well you keep your eyes fixed on a stationary target while your head is moving. To keep your vision trained on a stationary target while moving your head, you must move your eyes. It is this eye movement that is recorded and studied.

An abnormal test result shows a problem with the vestibulo-ocular reflex. One published study suggests that people with Meniere's disease have a specific test result, but auto-rotation testing is not generally used for that purpose.

Comparisons

Auto-rotation testing does not require a dedicated room or computerized "furniture" like the SHAT (rotary chair test). (It should be billed at a lower price.) Auto-rotation testing studies both horizontal and vertical head movement and also studies the vestibular-ocular reflex at higher speeds (which is probably more like the movement encountered in everyday life) than the rotary chair test. Auto-rotation testing is done quickly compared to most other vestibular tests. Many people consider it more comfortable than ENG testing.

After the Test

People sensitive to head movement or eye movement after head movement may have their symptoms temporarily stirred up by this test. Plan to have someone drive you home, or stay put until you are able to drive.

Computerized Dynamic Posturography (CDP)

This is a group of tests of the vestibulo-spinal reflex, which creates muscle movements necessary to maintain balance when you are standing or sitting. Computerized dynamic posturography (CDP) is also sometimes called dynamic posturography, moving platform posturography, dynamic computerized platform posturography, and platform posturography.

A computer creates all the changes experienced during the test and automatically records the body's responses.

Preparation

Because the testing equipment includes a harness to keep you from falling, wear shorts or slacks for the test. You will also be asked to remove your shoes and possibly your socks. Allow about an hour for the test.

Insurance/billing note: Some insurance companies will not pay for CDP testing. Check with your insurance company before scheduling the test. The testing center may also be able to give you a general idea about problems related to insurance. If you receive itemized bills, CDP testing may be charged in two or three parts: sensory organization test, motor coordination test, and pressure test.

What Is It Like?

Before beginning the test, you will be fitted with a harness similar to those worn by parachutists or rock climbers. (See Figure 16-5.) It will keep you from falling down if you have a loss of balance. You will be asked to stand quietly on a flat surface during the entire test and will be given instructions about when to open your eyes and when to close them. The surface under your feet will be still at times and will move at other times. The "wall" directly in front of you will be still and perfectly vertical at most times but will automatically move slightly at times.

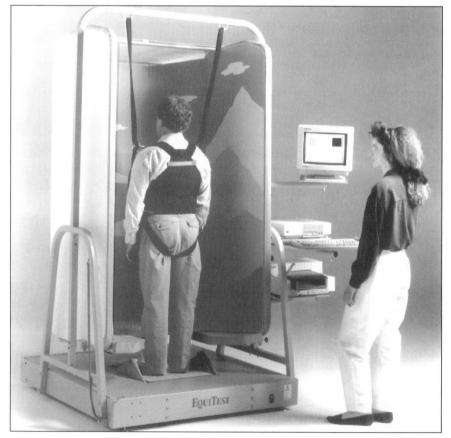

Figure 16-5: Computerized dynamic posturography. (Courtesy of NeuroCom International, Inc., Clackamas, Oregon.)

Sometimes a pressure test will be included in CDP testing. It involves inserting an ear piece into your ear, introducing positive and negative pressure, and measuring your movement or sway. This procedure is repeated with positive and negative pressure in each ear, one ear at a time.

What Does It Show?

CDP testing shows how well balance is maintained in response to various situations, such as when information is available from vision, proprioception, and the vestibular apparatus vs. when information is available from only two or only one of these systems or when the information from one or more is inaccurate. Information is unavailable or inaccurate when your eyes are closed, when the "wall" is moving, and when the surface under your feet is allowed to move.

Testing also measures muscle response to changing balance situations. Certain muscle "strategies" are used subconsciously and automatically to maintain balance, and these can also be assessed. Finally, CDP can measure balance response to increased and decreased pressure in each ear.

CDP may only indicate if a problem is present and not if the trouble is in the inner ear, nerve, or brain. A possible exception is pressure testing done one ear at a time; presumably, the pressure can affect only the middle ear and inner ear windows on the side being tested. No generally accepted CDP specifically diagnoses Meniere's disease.

Other Uses

Because this test shows muscle responses, some doctors use it not only to make a diagnosis but to determine if some type of physical therapy might help you and, if so, what type. The test can also be repeated from time to time to document changes in balance ability.

Comparisons

CDP is different from the other tests because it is done standing, does not use facial electrodes, tests body movement rather than eye movement, and usually involves no mental tasking or exercises. This test is the only computerized test discussed in this chapter that does not measure the VOR. Instead it looks at the vestibulo-spinal reflex (VSR) and the muscle movement it produces. CDP can also be used to develop specific physical therapy exercises that could be of benefit. (Physical therapy is generally more beneficial for people with inner ear problems other than Meniere's disease, but exceptions arise.)

After the Test

CDP should not cause any ill effects other than momentary spatial disorientation, confusion about your position in space, and possibly some fatigue. If this test sounds like something that would bother you, ask someone to drive you home from the test, or stay put until you are again able to drive.

Chapter 17

Miscellaneous Tests

Allergy Tests

Because allergies can cause symptoms resembling those of Meniere's disease, you may be referred to an allergist to determine if you have allergies. Allergy testing may involve having a blood test and/or allergy skin tests, and/or eliminating items from your diet or home environment.

No methods exist for directly testing someone for specific inner ear allergies. A positive allergy skin test does not necessarily mean that a substance is causing your apparent inner ear symptoms.

Who Is Tested?

Some doctors routinely have all their patients tested, while others may never look at the allergy possibility. People with a history of hay fever may have a greater chance of an allergy problem causing their symptoms. Some studies suggest that as many as one third of the people diagnosed with Meniere's disease also have an allergy.

MRI

In some ways a magnetic resonance imaging (MRI) scan is similar to an X-Ray since you are expected to be still during the test and since the final product looks like an X-Ray image. But there is one big difference: an MRI uses a magnetic field instead of X-Rays.

A brain MRI is not used to "find" Meniere's disease; it is used to look for brain abnormalities such as multiple sclerosis, stroke, and tumors. Some brain abnormalities can, on occasion, cause symptoms similar to those of Meniere's disease. Some doctors request an MRI almost automatically for people with vertigo, while others do so only if the symptoms and medical history point strongly toward the possibility of a brain problem.

Preparation

Before scheduling or going for an MRI, get written instructions from the staff of your doctor's office or the testing center and read them carefully. If you have any metal in your body, you **must** discuss this with the testing staff. Metal would include a cardiac pacemaker, orthopedic "pin," a Cody tack, shrapnel, coronary artery clips, any type of vascular clips, a vena caval umbrella, joint prosthesis, neurostimulator, orthodontics, insulin infusion pump, middle ear prosthesis, bullets, or small bits of metal that a metal worker might have picked up through his or her career. (The testing center should provide you with a more complete list of possible body metals.) If you have some type of medical implant, do not assume that anyone else knows about it. Ask and inform.

If you are prone to claustrophobia, discuss it with your doctor or the staff of the testing center. Some MRI machines are designed in an "open" fashion, but most of them are of the older, "closed" variety.

Special Precautions

This test cannot be stopped midway without interfering with the brain image it is creating. Use the restroom before beginning the test to avoid the problems a test stoppage would create.

Do not enter the MRI room with credit cards, an ATM card, debit card, or anything else with a magnetic coded strip on the back. Do not take computer disks into the MRI room; the magnetic field will erase all these things.

How Does an MRI Work?

This testing method is used to see soft tissue (not bones) using a large magnetic field instead of traditional X-Rays. The magnetic field causes the hydrogen ions of the body to change position; this causes the ions to give off radio waves. The radio waves are picked up by a receiver, and this information is sent to the computer, where an image is constructed.

What Is It Like?

You will be asked to arrive at the testing center early for any needed paperwork, to change your clothes, remove your jewelry, and to lock up your valuables. If you have any last minute questions, you should ask them before the test begins.

After telling you about the procedure, the MRI technician will have you lie down on a thin mattress, insert ear plugs, and in some testing centers, your head will be secured in one position with padding and a velcro strap to prevent head movement. You will then be slid into a doughnut-shaped opening at one end of the MRI machine. This machine does not move, and its opening does not change in any way during the test. The technician will be outside the room you are in and will be in voice contact with you during the entire test. Some machines have a mirror mounted above your head to allow you to see out into the room at all times. Many MRI testing places are also able to play music during the test.

You will be instructed to be absolutely still while the machine is working. While working, it makes a banging noise the ear plugs are meant to protect against. Do not speak with the technician while the machine is making a noise unless an emergency arises.

Many times an MRI test includes the use of a chemical called gadolinium, which will help identify any abnormal brain growths. The chemical will either be injected directly into a vein, or an IV will be started to give the drug. You may experience a brief burning sensation in the area of the injection or infusion, but it will quickly pass, and the injection causes no other sensations.

You will be in the machine about 30-45 minutes. The banging noise will occur only part of the time.

How much of the inner ear can be seen on a routine brain MRI? The interior cannot be seen at all. Even the outer shell may only be partially visible. See Figure 17-1.

Cochlea

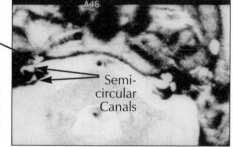

Figure 17-1: Magnetic resonance imaging (MRI) of the head. A cochlea and two semicircular canals are visible on the left.

Semi-circular Canals

Insurance note: If you must get prior approval from your insurance company, make sure you have it before going for this test. If a test must be done in an "approved" facility, make sure the MRI testing center is included on your insurance company's list. Another word of caution: an MRI machine located within an approved hospital could be owned and operated by a separate group or business that is not approved. Ask.

On occasion, your doctor might suggest a magnetic resonance angiography (MRA) test. It evaluates blood flow in the area tested. Taking an MRA test will not seem any different from taking an MRI.

X-Rays

X-rays cannot diagnose Meniere's disease. When X-rays are

requested, they are used to look for abnormal growths or fractures or to view the anatomy around the ear(s). Currently X-rays are not used frequently during the diagnosis of Meniere's disease. In someone with Meniere's disease, some characteristics of anatomy, such as the width of the vestibular aqueduct, may be different from normal. That difference is not generally used to make a diagnosis.

CT Scans

Some doctors will arrange for a computerized tomography (CT) scan of the temporal bone before doing certain inner ear surgeries.

Blood Tests

No blood test exists to detect the presence of Meniere's disease. However, your doctor may order a battery of blood tests anyway. The tests are usually done to look for specific conditions known to cause symptoms similar to Meniere's disease and to look at your general health. Specific blood tests for syphilis and thyroid disease are commonly done along with tests for anemia, abnormal blood sugar levels, abnormal mineral (electrolyte) levels, infections, elevated cholesterol, elevated triglycerides, and more.

In some areas of the country, a blood test for inner ear antigens may be done. This test, when positive, may point to an autoimmune reaction in the inner ear. Other blood tests, when positive, can point toward an autoimmune reaction occurring somewhere in the body, but these tests cannot identify the exact area(s) under attack.

ABR

The auditory brainstem response (ABR) test also examines hearing but cannot be used to "rule in" Meniere's disease. The ABR is also referred to as a "brainstem elicited response" that may be abbreviated as BER, BSER, BAER, and so on. The test is usually referred to as an *auditory brainstem response* by otolaryngologists and as a *brainstem elicited response* by neurologists.

The ABR is a sophisticated, computerized test of hearing. As sound makes its way to the brainstem (a part of the brain), it creates an electrical signal. This signal is recorded during the ABR and analyzed.

What Is It Like?

The test is done in a quiet area while you are comfortably seated or reclining. Sticky patches (electrodes) are placed on your head. You are asked to rest quietly while listening to the sounds introduced by headphones. You are not asked to respond.

What Does the ABR Show?

If hearing is abnormal, it shows where in the pathway the problem lies. This test is similar to an ECOG except that sound is tracked all the way into the brainstem, not just to the vestibulo-cochlear nerve.

Under certain circumstances, this test can indicate the presence of a tumor called an acoustic neuroma. Before the advent of the MRI, this was the test for acoustic neuroma (a benign tumor of the vestibular branch of the vestibulo-cochlear nerve).

Other Uses

The ABR test may also be used as an objective measurement of hearing. It can measure hearing in someone unable or unwilling to undergo a more routine hearing test.

This test is also used by some doctors to look for a condition sometimes called vascular compression.

Middle Ear Endoscopy

On rare occasions, a doctor may want to closely examine the middle ear for the cause of the symptoms. This minor surgical procedure can be done in the doctor's office.

What Is It Like?

A topical anesthetic is applied to the tympanic membrane, and a small incision is made through which an endoscope is inserted. The endoscope is a thin, lighted tube with appropriate wires and fibers. It lights the middle ear and sends an image back to the end of the scope the surgeon is staring into. The doctor looks at this as you might look into your camcorder and moves the end in the ear to allow him or her to look around. With the proper attachments, the endoscope can also be used to take pictures of the middle ear.

What Does the Endoscope Show?

The endoscope can reveal inflammation, scarring, infection, posssibly a perilymph fistula, and on rare occasion a growth called a cholesteatoma. (This growth is more common in someone who has had multiple middle ear infections.)

Other Uses

Some surgeons use an endoscope to view the middle ear before instilling certain medicines into it.

Pressure Testing

The observation that some people with Meniere's disease seem to experience improved hearing after being placed in a low pressure tank has been used as a treatment in Europe and Japan for a number of years.

It has also been suggested that a low pressure chamber might be used as a diagnostic tool. The thought is that if your hearing improves when you are placed in a low pressure chamber, you might have Meniere's disease.

Neither the pressure treatment nor the pressure test are universally accepted as worthwhile.

Chapter 18
Future Tests

The future should bring with it new and better tests, available on a large scale, to help in the diagnosis and treatment of inner ear problems.

"Functional" MRI may someday provide a method of determining hair cell and neural function for both hearing and balance.

It may also provide an objective test for the presence of tinnitus or for visualizing Reissner's membrane (the membrane thought to be displaced and broken in Meniere's disease).

Also, because the two inner ear fluids have different chemical compositions that may become discernible via MRI, the test may be used to study these fluids in living people and to see if symptoms are caused by the mixing of these two fluids.

Vestibular evoked response testing, the vestibular equivalent of the ECOG or ABR, may become possible in humans and allow new tests of vestibular function.

Advances in molecular biology, so helpful in other fields, should begin to benefit otology also, especially for inherited disorders.

Tests of vestibular apparatus structures such as the otolithic organs may become available outside research labs.

Blood tests may become possible for inner ear antigens and other substances that can potentially cause hearing loss and vestibular symptoms related to immune disorders.

References

Here is a list of books and articles used in preparation of this and the preceding chapters on testing:

Arenberg, I.K. *Dizziness and Balance Disorders: An Interdisciplinary Approach to Diagnosis and Treatment.* New York: Kugler, 1993.

Baloh, R.W., and Halmagyi, G.M. *Disorders of the Vestibular System.* New York: Oxford University Press, 1996.

Baloh, R.W., and Honrubia, V. *Clinical Neurophysiology of the Vestibular System.* Philadelphia: F.A. Davis Company, 1990.

Black, F.O. "Vestibulospinal Function Assessment by Moving Platform Posturography." *American Journal of Otology*, 39-45, 1985.

Booth, J.B. *Scott-Brown's Otolaryngology, Vol. 3, Otology,* Fifth Edition. London: Butterworth's, 1987.

Cass, S.P., and Furman, J.M. "Medications and Their Effects on Vestibular Function Testing," http://www.icsmedical.com/november1993.htm. Dec. 3, 1997.

Cevette, M.J., Puetz, B., Marion, M.S., Wertz, M.L., and Muenter, M.D. "Aphysiologic Performance on Dynamic Posturography," *Otolaryngology Head and Neck Surgery,* 112:676-688, 1995.

Filipo, R., and Barbara, M. "Meniere's Disease—Perspective in the '90s." *Proceedings of the Third International Symposium on Meniere's Disease, Rome, Italy,* October 20-23, 1993. New York: Kugler Publications, 1994.

Green J.D., Blum., D.J., and Harner, S.G. "Longitudinal Follow-Up of Patients with Meniere's Disease." *Otolaryngology—Head and Neck Surgery,* 104:783-788, 1991.

Harvey, S.A., and Wood, D.J. "The Oculocephalic Response in the Evaluation of the Dizzy Patient." *Laryngoscope,* 106:6-9, 1996.

Hoffman, D.L., O'Leary, D.P., and Munjack, D.J. "Autorotation Test Abnormalities of the Horizontal and Vertical Vestibulo-Ocular Reflexes in Panic Disorder." *Otolaryngology—Head and Neck Surgery,* 110:259-269, 1994.

Honrubia, V. "Contemporary Vestibular Function Testing: Accomplishments and Future Perspectives." *Otolaryngology — Head and Neck Surgery,* 112:64-77, 1995.

Jacobson, G.P., Newman, C.W., and Kartush, J.M. *Handbook of Balance Function Testing.* St Louis: Mosby Year Book, 1993.

Kitahara, M., Kodama, A., Ozawa, H., and Izukura, H. "Pressure Test for the Diagnosis of Meniere's Disease." *Acta Otolaryngologica, Supplement,* 510:107-110, 1994.

Koyunca, M., Mason, S.M., and Saunders, M.W. "Electrocochleography in Endolymphatic Hydrops Using Tone-Pip and Click Stimuli." *Clinical Otolaryngology,* 19:73-78, 1994.

Lee, C.S., Paparella, M.M., Margolis, R.H., and Le, C. "Audiological Profiles and Meniere's Disease." *Ear, Nose and Throat Journal,* 74(8):527-532, 1995.

Merchant, S.N., Rauch, S.D., and Nadol, J.B. "Meniere's Disease." *European Archives of Otorhinolaryngology,* 252:63-75,1995.

Nashner, L.M., and Peters, J.F. "Dynamic Posturography in the Diagnosis and Management of Dizziness and Balance Disorders." *Neurological Clinics*, 8(2):331-349, 1990.

National Institute on Deafness and Other Communication Disorders. "What Is Meniere's Disease?" http://www.nih.gov/nidcd/meniere.htm. July 25, 1997.

Ng, M., Davis, L.L., and O'Leary, D.P. "Autorotation Test of the Horizontal Vestibulo-Ocular Reflex in Meniere's Disease." *Otolaryngology—Head and Neck Surgery*, 109:399-412, 1993.

Northern, J.L. *Hearing Disorders*. Second edition. Boston: Allyn and Bacon, 1984.

Poe, D.S., Rebeiz, E.E., Pankratov, M.M., and Shapshay, S.M. "Transtympanic Endoscopy of the Middle Ear." *Laryngoscope*, 102:993-996, 1992.

Pfaltz, C.R. *Controversial Aspects of Meniere's Disease*. New York: Thieme, Inc., 1986.

Rahn, J.E. *Ears, Hearing, and Balance*. New York: Atheneum, 1984.

Rosenberg, S.I., Silverstein, H., Willcox, T.O., and Gordon, M.A. "Endoscopy in Otology and Neurotology." *American Journal of Otology*, 15(2):168-171, 1994.

Shepard, N.T., and Telian, S.A. *Practical Management of the Balance Disorder Patient*. San Diego: Singular Publishing Group, Inc., 1996.

Therapeutics and Technology Assessment Subcommittee. "Assessment: Posturography." *Neurology*, 43:1261-1264, 1993.

Van de Heyning, P.H., Kingma, H., and Claes, J. "Introduction: Meniere's Disease: State of the Art." *Acta Otolaryngologica, Supplement*, 526:4, 1997.

Von Gierke, H.E., et al. "Evaluation of Tests for Vestibular Function." *Aviation, Space, and Environmental Medicine*, 63(2, supplement):A1-A34, 1992.

Watanabe, T.K. "Nystagmus During an Acute Attack of Meniere's Disease." http://www.icsmedical.com/march1996.htm. Dec. 3, 1997.

Part IV: Treatment

Though no cure is known for Meniere's disease, many treatments have been reported to stop or to mitigate some of its symptoms in some people at least some of the time.

Chapter 19

Treatment— Introduction

In general, the treatment goal for any disease is to effect a cure. For Meniere's disease there is no "cure" nor any means of reversing its damage. However, Meniere's symptoms can often be "controlled," and many of them may disappear on their own. While "cure" may not be a reasonable goal, it is reasonable to expect your doctor to address your needs for safety and comfort.

Treatments aim at preventing attacks, stopping nausea and vomiting, relieving attacks, blocking the symptoms between attacks, making tinnitus more bearable, and relieving hearing loss or deafness through the use of hearing aids or cochlear implants.

Many treatments exist for Meniere's disease, but no single treatment helps everyone. Unfortunately the most common way of finding a successful treatment is by trial and error. If a treatment works, you can stick with it; if it does not, many more are available. Don't give up.

A Quick Word About Surgery

Many textbooks and other sources of Meniere's disease information focus heavily on surgical treatments. When looking at "ear" textbooks, you might get the impression that surgery is the most common or important treatment for Meniere's disease and, for that matter, other inner ear vestibular problems. In fact, this is not the case and never has been. Surgery is reserved for use when all other treatments have failed and when someone is so severely affected by the symptoms that he or she cannot function in a reasonably normal way in everyday life. Most people with Meniere's disease will never require surgery for symptom control.

The reason that so much textbook information exists about Meniere's surgery is not that surgery is generally important in the treatment of Meniere's disease but the fact that surgery is technically demanding and needs a lot of explaining. Surgery may relieve vertigo in some cases, but it is generally acknowledged that surgery cannot be relied on to improve tinnitus, hearing loss, or aural fullness.

Choosing a Treatment

The treatment options your doctor suggests to you may depend on many things, including the following:

• your age and physical condition
• your level of hearing
• the amount of your disability
• your doctor's opinion of what might be causing your symptoms
• your doctor's experience with treating and observing patients like you
• the demands upon your physician
• your financial or insurance situation
• whether one or both ears are affected
• what symptoms you have, their strength, and your reaction to them
• what your doctor learned in medical school and during residency training about Meniere's disease

Because the cause of Meniere's disease is unknown, some doctors will begin by using several treatments simultaneously. This method is sometimes called the "shotgun approach." The idea is to achieve success quickly. However, if improvement occurs, it may be hard to tell which treatment worked.

Why Is Finding an Effective Treatment Difficult?

Finding an effective treatment is difficult for many reasons. The following quotations may shed light on the problems:

> "Another factor to be considered, especially when any particular form of treatment is being assessed, is the natural tendency of the disease towards spontaneous remission, and it is important to guard against attributing such a remission to a successful response to treatment."
>
> —T.E. Cawthorne,
> *Journal of Laryngology and Otology*, 1943

> "The criteria of the diagnosis are also loose and what may be considered as Meniere's disease by one may be denied categorically by another clinician. The greatest controversy exists in the therapeutic efforts. A bewildering number of concepts and methods have been suggested, tried, and praised as the best answers in solving the problem until the next claim of success shatters the popularity of earlier allegations. All the published ideas, regimens, and techniques have one signifi-

cant feature in common. They all claim success but not in 100 percent of the cases. Recovery varies from about 60 percent to 80 percent."

—N. Torok, *Laryngoscope,* 1977

More reasons for this difficulty in finding a single effective treatment are as follows:

- The structure and function of the inner ear are difficult to study and not totally understood.
- The changes within the inner ear that precipitate the attack symptoms and other symptoms are not well understood.
- The cause or event that puts Meniere's disease into motion is unknown.
- The motion/gravity sensing areas of the inner ear cannot be directly viewed or their function directly measured.
- Meniere's disease does not follow a set pattern; it ebbs and flows randomly, and this makes scientific study difficult.
- Only a few treatments have been subjected to controlled human studies.
- It's difficult to study enough people undergoing any particular treatment for the results to be meaningful.
- Treatments can't usually be evaluated objectively. The evaluations usually depend upon people with Meniere's disease saying how they feel before and after treatment.
- Meniere's disease may not be a single disease; it may be many conditions with similar symptoms. These different conditions may require different treatments.

What Is the Most Common Approach?

In the United States, the most common treatment is the use of both a low sodium diet and a diuretic in an attempt to decrease the amount of endolymph in the inner ear by decreasing fluids throughout the body. The idea behind this is that excess endolymph is thought to be the problem in Meniere's disease and that reducing this fluid by decreasing fluids throughout the body may improve symptoms.

Table 19-1, on the following page, lists methods or means that have been used to treat Meniere's disease. They will be further examined in the next chapters of this book.

Why Not Just Reduce Excess Endolymph?

It is not known for certain that this is the actual problem in

Table 19-1: Treatment Methods

Alternative Therapies

acupuncture	craniosacral	naturopathy
chiropractic	homeopathy	Therapak II

Dietary Changes

low sodium diet	avoiding "problem" items

Drugs

adrenergics	betahistine	oil of primrose
aminoglycosides or	calcium channel	sedatives
chemical destruction	blockers	steroids
anesthetics	diuretics	vasodilators
antihistamines	ginger root	vasoconstrictors
anticholinergics	ginseng	vitamins
antidepressants	histamines	

Others

overpressure	physical therapy	vestibular
psychological	t'ai chi	rehabilitation
treatment	underpressure	

Smoking Cessation

Stress Control

aromatherapy	massage	relaxation exercises
biofeedback	meditation	therapeutic touch
hypnosis	yoga	

Surgery

Meniere's disease, and even if it is, reducing the fluid and its pressure is easier said than done. Diet therapies, medications (both water pills and circulation drugs), and a surgical procedure (endolymphatic shunt) are meant to reduce the amount of endolymph, but no method is entirely successful.

Disclaimer

VEDA and the author do not mean to endorse or disavow the many treatments mentioned in this book. The treatments mentioned here have already been discussed in scientific and civilian journals, magazines, newsletters, and other publications. We have included them so that you can learn about their large number and great diversity. Some of these treatments have been widely used in the United States, where this book was written and published; others have not.

What treatment, if any, you choose should depend upon consultations with your physician.

References

Cawthorne, T.E. "The Treatment of Meniere's Disease." *Journal of Laryngology and Otology,* 58:363-371, 1943.

Torok, N. "The Old and New in Meniere's Disease." *Laryngoscope,* 87:1870-77, 1977.

Chapter 20

Diet

No standard Meniere's disease diet exists. Doctors disagree about which, if any, diet is valuable. Your doctor (based on his or her experience and beliefs) may recommend that you change your diet. The more common diets try to do one or more of the following:

- reduce the amount of endolymph
- improve blood supply to the inner ear
- keep the amount of endolymph in the inner ear from fluctuating too much
- eliminate foods that may directly affect the inner ear

Reducing Endolymph

A low-sodium diet is probably the most commonly recommended and the oldest in use for Meniere's disease. As with all other treatments for Meniere's disease, some people following it will improve and others will not.

Low-Sodium Diets in General

The aim of a low-sodium diet is to reduce the overabundance of endolymph within the inner ear. The sodium content in the diet is cut back in the hope that the amount of water in the body, including the inner ear, will decrease.

A reduced sodium diet usually asks you to consume less than a certain amount of sodium per day. The sodium weight limit is generally listed in milligrams or grams and varies from 1,000 to 4,000 milligrams (or 1 to 4 grams). Some doctors may also refer to this kind of diet as "low-salt" or "salt-poor." On this kind of diet, you will be asked to keep score of your total intake of sodium per each 24 hours. To be accurate, you must count the sodium in everything you eat and everything you drink and any sodium you ingest from other sources such as vitamin pills and drinking water. Simply limiting the salt you add to your food does not make your diet a low-sodium diet; you must count all sodium.

Note on metric measurements: Milligrams, grams, and kilograms are metric measurements of weight. There are 1,000 milligrams (mg) in a gram (gm) and 1,000 grams in a kilogram (kg). One kilogram weighs approximately 2.2 pounds, and one pound weighs approximately 454 grams. A 1,000 mg (milligram) diet is the same as a 1 gram diet.

Why are the measurements metric? The English system is not good for expressing small weights in a clear and memorable way. For example, a 1 gram diet would be a .0022026 pound diet.

Sodium is a chemical needed for normal water balance throughout the body and for nerve function. To have a normal amount of body water, you must have a normal amount of sodium. (In the body, water is used to dissolve things, to provide a place for chemical reactions to occur, for lubrication, for transport, and to help body temperature regulation. The sodium we are speaking of here is the dissolved, ionized form, not pure metallic sodium.)

The chemical abbreviation for sodium is Na. Sodium, chemically combined with other substances, is a natural constituent of some foods and is added to many others in the form of table salt. Table salt is more formally called sodium chloride (a chemical compound of sodium and chlorine), and its chemical abbreviation is NaCl. One teaspoon of NaCl contains 2,396 mg of sodium.

The minimum daily healthy intake of sodium for good health is 500 mg (although as low as 100 mg may be okay for some people). The daily sodium value used in food labeling in the United States is 2,400 mg, set by the National Research Council. The average person in the U.S. takes in around 4,000 to 6,000 mg in a day.

Note about sodium: If you would like to see how sodium chloride can manipulate water, place a fresh peeled carrot in a plastic bag, shake on some salt, and set aside for a few hours. Later, when you return to this bag, you will find water in it. This water was "pulled" out of the carrot's cells by the sodium in table salt.

Sodium Information

The only way to know the sodium contents of fresh vegetables, fruits, meats, fish, etc., is to look them up in a reference book or list. Your local library should have a guide to low-sodium eating including menus and recipes. The *VEDA Low-Salt Cookbook* is available from The Vestibular Disorders Association (VEDA). Bookstores in your area should also have books covering this topic. The American Heart Association has many publications on low-sodium diets.

If you have a water softening system, check the documentation for the amount of sodium it puts into your water.

Note: The University of Iowa Press publishes a 100-page book by Brian F. McCabe, M.D., with lists of food sodium amounts and calories. This book could easily fit into your pocket or purse. Although its title is *Low-Salt Diet for Meniere's Disease,* it is primarily a list of the sodium content of various foods and does not include recipes or sample menus.

This book is available through the Department of Otolaryngology—Head and Neck Surgery at the University of Iowa Hospitals and Clinics, Iowa City, Iowa 52242 for $5, which includes shipping and handling.

Food From Stores and Restaurants

Most foods in the U.S. come with nutritional information somewhere on their packaging. Look for the amount of sodium listed with all the other nutritional information. Don't look for it in the list of ingredients (which is separate on the label from the nutrition facts), and don't be fooled by advertisements saying "no salt added;" this does not necessarily mean that the product is low in sodium.

When you look at the label, check for two things, the serving size and the milligrams of sodium per serving. Sometimes the product label will define a serving as a portion that is much smaller than the one you are going to eat. Beware of counting too low when this happens.

Establishments such as McDonald's and Burger King have nutritional information about their food posted or available upon request. Some reference books include the sodium content of meals at many large chain restaurants. You can call other restaurants and ask about the sodium content of items on their menus.

Fast food restaurants, generally speaking, serve food high in sodium.

General Guidelines About Sodium

Table salt, sea salt, onion salt, garlic salt, celery salt, and MSG (monosodium glutamate) are all high in sodium.

Foods that have not been processed generally have a low sodium content. (If you ate only unprocessed food and did not add any salt, your sodium intake would be around 500 mg a day.)

Processed foods generally have a high amount of sodium, and the sodium content increases with the degree of processing. For example, here's a comparison of the sodium content of three ounces of three kinds of roast beef, from least processed to most processed: cooked, 54 mg; canned and corned, 855 mg; chipped, 2,949 mg.

Highly processed dairy foods like cheese have a large sodium content, and those less processed, like milk, have moderate amounts of sodium.

"Snack foods" such as potato chips, cheese nachos, pretzels, little sausages, pizza, crackers, salted nuts, and buttered and/or salted popcorn generally have a high amount of sodium.

Some ethnic cuisines have a higher concentration of sodium than others.

Most pre-cooked, pre-packaged meals like pot pies and pizza are high-sodium foods. Sauces of all sorts are usually high in sodium (soy, Worcestershire, catsup, mustard, fish, teriyaki, barbeque, etc.). This is also true of most salad dressings.

Tomato products such as catsup, tomato sauce, tomato puree, tomato paste, and spaghetti sauce are typically high in sodium.

Table 20-1: Some Low-Sodium Foods

fish that has not been cured, smoked, pickled, salted, or cooked or processed in any way that adds salt

fresh fruit

fresh vegetables

many frozen vegetables

meats that have not been cured, smoked, pickled, salted, or cooked or processed in any way that adds salt

noodles, couscous, and pasta cooked without salt

rice

Table 20-2: Some Processed Foods High In Sodium

anything pickled	ham
bacon	"lunch" meats
breaded fish fillets	mayonnaise
canned soups	pickles (all types)
canned tomato juice	refried beans
canned vegetables	sausages
corned beef	seafood sauce
dry packed soups	turkeys of the butterball type

Planning Meals in Advance

To help with your low-sodium diet, plan your meals for a day in your usual manner. Find the sodium contents of the food for those meals, and add them up for each meal and for the day. Make sure you are using the serving size used by your reference book or defined on the packaging of the processed foods.

Your daily goal is to make your total sodium intake equal to the amount suggested by your doctor and for each of your meals to be roughly equal in sodium content. If the initial menu exceeds the goal, substitute lower sodium items or change the serving amounts until you arrive at the goal. Some people find small food scales helpful in determining the weights of different foods. (You can also use a postal scale.)

Spread your sodium intake over the entire day. Avoid a pattern in which you skip breakfast, then eat a lunch with only 150 mg of sodium, and then have an evening meal that includes 1,000 mg. Try to keep the sodium totals about the same for all three meals.

Finding Substitutes

You will find many herbs, spices, and flavors to try instead of salt: oregano, garlic, lemon juice, cinnamon, curry, ginger, mustard powder, paprika, parsley, thyme, and nutmeg. Many potassium-based salts can replace sodium salt (table salt). Flavor French fries with malt vinegar instead of salt and catsup. Also, some processed foods have a low sodium content, but you must look for them on the shelves at your local grocery store and at health food stores.

Table 20-3: Salt Substitutes	
Adolph's salt substitute	NoSalt
Co-salt	seasoned NoSalt
Mrs. Dash and all varieties	nu-salt

This juggling act of preparing a menu will be difficult at first, but once you are familiar with the sodium contents of your favorite foods, it will become easier.

Can Anything Bad Happen Because of a Low-Sodium Diet?

There's a small chance that your blood sodium level will fall below normal, particularly any time you sweat profusely, vomit, or get diarrhea. Also, people with low blood pressure may see it go even lower, possibly leading to lightheadedness and faintness. No statistics are available for the occurrence of these problems, but the incidence is probably low.

Decreasing Endolymph Fluctuation

Another type of diet, based on six small meals a day instead of the U.S. average of three, is meant to prevent large fluctuations in fluid levels and therefore in endolymph levels throughout the day. This diet aims at keeping the amount of sodium and sugar entering the blood stream similar at each meal and snack.

The six-meal diet may be prescribed in addition to a low-sodium diet. In that case, you would follow the instructions for the low-sodium diet but divide the sodium intake into six roughly equal parts.

Improving the Inner Ear's Blood Supply

Some doctors feel you may be able to increase the supply of blood to your inner ears by eliminating certain items from your diet. They feel food and drink containing caffeine may cause the blood vessels to constrict (get smaller) and decease the amount of blood getting into and out of the inner ears. These items include coffee, tea, and colas such as Coke, Pepsi, RC Cola, generic colas, Mountain Dew, Dr. Pepper, Tab, Mello Yellow, Mr. Pibb, and any other soft drinks containing caffeine. You may also be told to eliminate chocolate, which contains a caffeine-like substance, and any drugs that contain caffeine. (Over-the-counter drugs, particularly analgesics and anti-sleep drugs, often contain caffeine.) A low-cholesterol diet may be suggested at times as well.

Avoiding Things That Can Directly Affect the Inner Ear

Allergens

If your doctor suspects a food allergy to be the cause of your problem, he or she may prescribe a special diet that limits or eliminates the problem food(s).

A rotation diet is sometimes used in which you eat the problem food(s) only once every four or more days.

Alcohol

Alcoholic beverages may cause a problem for some people with Meniere's disease, for any of the following reasons:

- Taking any sedative or depressive drug, including alcohol, will decrease your balance ability because your level of alertness will be lowered.
- Alcohol will cause temporary changes in the density of your inner ear fluids, and this will change the way your inner ear senses gravity and movement.
- Alcohol causes many drugs (like diazepam, meclizine, and similar drugs) used to treat the symptoms of Meniere's disease to be stronger than normal.
- Alcohol stops the action of the naturally occurring antidiuretic hormone (ADH), causing dehydration. This may cause endolymph levels to fluctuate enough to create a problem in some people.

A Final Word

If your doctor suggests a diet, try not to think of it as inherently negative. In general these are diets most health organizations would characterize as very healthy. If a diet change eliminates your violent vertigo, it will become much easier to like.

If you can control your symptoms with dietary changes, you will be using the cheapest treatment available with the lowest risk to you.

References

Dudek, S.G. *Nutrition: Handbook for Nursing Practice.* Second edition. Philadelphia: JB Lippincott, 1993.

Nelson, J.K., Moxness, K.E., Jensen, M.D., and Gastineau, C.F. *Mayo Clinic Diet Manual: A Handbook of Nutrition Practices.* Seventh edition. St. Louis: Mosby, 1994.

Sizer, F.A., and Whitney, E.N. *Hamilton and Whitney's Nutrition: Concepts and Controversies.* New York: West Publishing Company, 1994.

Wardlaw, G.M., Insel, P.M., and Seyler, M.F. *Contemporary Nutrition: Issues and Insights.* Second edition. St. Louis: Mosby, 1994.

Chapter 21

Drugs in General

Y ou should not be fearful of using drugs for Meniere's disease or any other condition, but you should respect their power. (This applies to over-the-counter drugs, herbs, and vitamins, as well as prescription drugs.) Drugs can do a lot of good, but they can also cause harm. Some bad results from drug therapy such as an allergic reaction probably can't be prevented, but other bad results can be avoided by following some rules:

- If you have allergic reactions to anything, wear a medic-alert kind of necklace or bracelet listing the substances you must avoid. (You can write to a company called MedicAlert at 2323 Colorado Ave., Turlock, CA 95382, for details, or call them at 1-800-763-3428.) Also, you should mention the substances you must avoid to every health-care professional you visit as a patient. Never assume that the doctor or nurse or other health-care professional already knows about your allergies.

- You should also wear a medic-alert kind of necklace or bracelet if you:
  - are taking a drug that should not be stopped suddenly
  - are on a special diet
  - have a hearing loss
  - take a drug called an MAO inhibitor
  - have any serious problems such as heart, lung, liver, or kidney disease
  - have glaucoma
  - have an enlarged prostate

- When you are getting a prescription from your doctor, make sure you know what the drug is, what it is supposed to do, how to take it, how much to take, when to take it, what changes you should report to the doctor if they occur, and what drugs and other substances it interacts with. (Most drugs, when combined with certain other drugs and substances, can cause effects different from the effects they cause by themselves.)

- Make a list of all your medications (including generic and trade names), when you take them, how much you take, the name of the doctor who prescribed them, and how long you have been taking them. Keep a copy of the list at home and another with you at all times.

- When you see them, review your medications list with your doctor(s) or any other health care providers giving you prescriptions or treatments.
- If you take more than one drug, make sure you are taking the right one at the right time for the right thing. Check the label each time to verify you have the correct one.
- Store your drugs in a dark, dry place with a temperature between 59 and 86 degrees for pills and below 77 degrees for suppositories. **(Don't store them in your bathroom; the hot air and humidity can alter them.)**
- Pills and suppositories can change in heat. Don't leave them in a car, particularly when the sun is out and the air temperature is warm.
- When you have to take a pill (tablet, capsule, or caplet), take it with a full glass of water unless instructed otherwise. Also, when possible, sit up for a while after swallowing a pill to help it get to your stomach.
- To avoid confusion and protect your medicine from light, keep your medicine in its original container.
- If any of the instructions on the medication's label are changed later, note the change and the date of change on the label, or attach a separate note to the medicine container.
- Get all of your drugs from the same pharmacy. Always ask if any new drugs you are planning to take are compatible with the older ones; this includes over-the-counter medications and any other drugs you are taking. (If you get drugs from several places, the pharmacists will not know all the drugs you are taking and cannot automatically check for possible drug conflicts.)
- Don't crush pills or open capsules unless you have been told it is okay for that particular medicine. The pill's packaging can affect where and how the contents are released into your body.
- If you have small children living with you or visiting, be careful where you store your medicines, and use child-proof caps. If you visit someone with small children, keep your medications where the children can't find them.
- If you think there is a problem with any of your medications or that you are having a problem caused by them, tell your doctor(s) and keep on telling them until you feel your concerns have been heard and addressed in some fashion. If you believe a medicine is causing a problem and a specialist has not listened to your concerns, try seeing your primary care doctor (family doctor) and discuss the situation with him or her. You can also discuss your medications and problems with your pharmacist and ask her or him to talk to your doctor.

Getting Drug Information

You can get reliable drug information from the doctor prescribing it or from the pharmacist dispensing it.

Bookstores and/or libraries have many excellent drug guides written for the public.

People who want more in-depth information can look through a nursing pharmacology textbook; these usually explain pertinent structure and function and are written for nursing students just out of high school. Many community colleges offer nursing courses, and their textbooks should be available in the school's library.

If you want even more information, you can try a pharmacology book like Goodman and Gilman's *The Pharmacological Basis of Therapeutics* or Katzung's *Basic and Clinical Pharmacology*, written for doctors, or Hansten and Horn's *Drug Interactions: Analysis and Management*. Texts like these assume that the reader has a solid grasp of medical terminology, and anatomy and physiology.

Generic Names; Trade Names

Drugs often have two different names, *generic* and *trade*. The generic name for a medicine is the one all drug companies can use to refer to a medication because the name is not owned by anyone. It might be considered the more "scientific" name and the one more difficult to pronounce, spell, and remember. When you choose a generic drug, you will probably get a brand made by a company other than the company that first marketed the drug.

The trade name is a medication name owned by a specific company. Trade names are usually shorter and easier to spell and remember than the generic drug names. Sometimes the name describes the use of the drug in some way. One popular inner ear drug called meclizine (generic name), is called Antivert (trade name) by the company that sells it.

Throughout this book, drugs will be referred to in a standard manner. The first letter in the generic name, as in meclizine, will be lowercase (unless appearing as the first letter in a sentence), and the first letter in a trade name will be uppercase, as in Antivert.

Athletes and Forbidden Drugs

The National Collegiate Athletic Association (NCAA) and the United States Olympic Committee (USOC) have rules forbidding the use of certain drugs by the athletes they represent. Drugs sometimes used to treat Meniere's disease may violate NCAA or USOC rules. These "banned" drugs include all diuretics (bumetanide, furosemide, acetazolamide, hydrochlorothiazide, etc.) and most steroids (prednisone, prenisolone, dexamethasone, cortisone, etc.).

References

_____. *Consumer Guide to Prescription Drugs.* Illinois: Publications International, Ltd., 1995.

_____. *The PDR Family Guide to Prescription Drugs.* Montvale, NJ: Medical Economics, 1995.

Griffith, H.W. *Complete Guide to Prescription and Non-Prescription Drugs.* Sixth edition. The Body Press, 1989.

Long, J.W., and Rybacki, J.J. *The Essential Guide to Prescription Drugs.* New York: Harper Perennial, 1994.

Silverman, H.M. *The Pill Book.* Seventh edition. New York: Bantam Books, 1996.

Wilson, B.A., Shannon, M.T., and Stang, C.L. *Nurses' Drug Guide 1993.* Norwalk: Appleton and Lange, 1993.

Chapter 22
Diuretics

Diuretics, commonly known as water pills, are used in Meniere's disease in an effort to reduce the amount of endolymph in the membranous labyrinth. The endolymph, the fluid in the endolymphatic space of the inner ear, is produced by cells in the walls of the scala media of the cochlea. The mechanism is similar to the one used by the kidney to exchange water and salt from blood to the urine. Diuretics, which reduce the amount of water throughout the body, are believed to exert the same effect in the inner ear. Diuretics from many drug families can be used for this purpose.

All diuretics work in the groups of kidney cells called nephrons that form urine. These drugs increase the amount of water leaving the body by sending more sodium into the urine. Each diuretic family works in a different area of the nephron and has somewhat different effects from the other families.

Diuretics are grouped into four categories or families in this chapter:
• thiazide diuretics
• potassium-sparing diuretics
• carbonic anhydrase inhibitors
• loop or high-ceiling diuretics

Although these drugs have different names and belong to different groups, they have many things in common.

• All diuretics in these four groups are related to "sulfa" drugs with the exception of one, ethacrynic acid (Edecrin). A potential for allergic reaction to all these sulfa relatives exists in individuals allergic to any of the sulfa drugs.

• Dehydration is a possible consequence from all of these drugs. Ask your doctor how many glasses of water you should drink throughout the day. A low sodium level can also occur when you use a diuretic. If you experience lightheadedness, muscle cramps, abdominal cramps, weakness, fatigue, tingling, or pins and needles sensations, report this to your doctor's office.

• Loss of potassium can occur when you take thiazide diuretics, carbonic anhydrase inhibitors, or loop diuretics. Many individuals will require supplemental potassium in pill, liquid, or powder form, while others only need to eat foods high in potassium when taking diuretics. Loss of potassium is not a major feature of the potassium-sparing diuretics like Maxzide and Dyazide.

Thiazide Diuretics

(Thiazide is the commonly used name, but benzothiazide is the proper name.)

Thiazide diuretics cause the kidneys to reduce the amount of sodium, chlorides, and magnesium in the blood stream, and they also lead to a reduction in potassium levels. Because of this, the potassium levels in the blood should be watched.

These diuretics also cause the kidneys to hang on to calcium and uric acid more than usual and increase blood sugar levels, particularly in individuals with diabetes mellitus.

Hydrochlorothiazide (HCTZ) is an example of a thiazide diuretic.

Coping Tip

If they upset your stomach by themselves, you can take thiazide diuretics with food or milk.

Potassium-Sparing Diuretics

Potassium-sparing diuretics are drugs that send only sodium into the urine and do not work by sending potassium into the urine; therefore they spare potassium. They actually hang on to potassium more than occurs under normal circumstances. The drugs in this category most frequently used to treat Meniere's disease are combinations of two drugs; they are therefore called combination drugs. Triamterene (Dyrenium), a potassium-sparing diuretic, is added to hydrochlorothiazide (HCTZ) to make the combination drugs Maxzide and Dyazide.

Possible Side Effects

Potassium-sparing diuretics can cause all the problems of other diuretics **but do not usually lower blood potassium levels.**

Warning about hyperkalemia: These drugs carry one warning in the 1998 *Physician's Desk Reference* (PDR). Abnormal elevation of serum potassium levels (hyperkalemia) can occur with all potassium-conserving diuretic combinations. Hyperkalemia is more likely to occur in patients with renal impairment, patients with diabetes (even without evidence of renal impairment), or elderly or severely ill patients. Since uncorrected hyperkalemia may be fatal, serum potassium levels must be monitored at frequent intervals (especially in patients taking these drugs for the first time), when dosages are changed, or with any illness that may influence renal function.

Carbonic Anhydrase Inhibitors

The drugs in this family inhibit an enzyme, carbonic anhydrase, and cause the kidneys to reduce the amount of sodium (Na+) ions in the blood stream along with potassium (K+) ions and bicarbonate (HCO_3-) ions.

One of the more common of these drugs is acetazolamide (Diamox).

Possible Side Effects

Numbness, burning and/or tingling of the lips, mouth, arms, and/or legs, are somewhat common and are usually not indications for stopping the drug but should be reported to the doctor's office as a precaution.

Coping Tip

Adequate intake of fluids is important to protect against the formation of kidney stones. These drugs should be taken with food and water to avoid stomach irritation.

Loop or High-Ceiling Diuretics

These drugs are the most potent of the diuretics. They also are the most likely to cause problems such as dehydration, decreased blood pressure, and mineral (electrolyte) imbalance. Not only do these diuretics cause the kidneys to reduce the amount of sodium in the blood stream, they also lead to a reduction in potassium levels.

Two common loop diuretics are furosemide (Lasix) and bumetanide (Bumex).

Possible Side Effects

The most common serious problem is a decreased potassium level that could cause muscle spasms.

On rare occasion, these drugs can cause inner ear poisoning (called ototoxicity) resulting in hearing loss. This loss can be permanent if you are taking a loop diuretic plus an aminoglycoside antibiotic or cisplatin, a chemotherapy drug. (See Chapter 34, "Preservation, Protection" for more information about ototoxicity.) It occurs most frequently in individuals with decreased or poor renal (kidney) function and those taking aminoglycoside antibiotics. It is not known if this effect occurs more frequently in individuals with inner ear damage.

Coping Tip

If you are taking a loop diuretic, you should be particularly careful about getting up from a sitting or lying position, or while standing for long periods, or during hot weather. These are situations in which the dehydrating effects and the lower blood pressure caused by these drugs are most likely to be felt.

Frequently Asked Questions

Why can't I just decrease my sodium intake and skip the diuretic?

Reduction of dietary sodium content is a slower method for decreasing body fluids in general. It is also difficult to maintain a low-sodium diet at all times and prevent the amount of fluid and sodium fluctuation that occurs when you eat two or three times per day. A diuretic can work faster and prevent some of the fluctuating. If you would prefer to rely solely on dietary controls, discuss this with your doctor.

What does sodium do in the body?

It is used in water balance and movement, fluid pressure regulation, nerve function, muscle function, and it helps transport glucose and other nutrients within the body.

How do I know if I am becoming dehydrated?

The signs and symptoms are non-specific. They do not automatically point to dehydration. They can be the symptoms for many other things, and a diagnosis is not usually made from the symptoms alone. The signs and symptoms include dry mouth, cotton feeling mouth, thirst, headache, dry and/or flushed skin, decreased amount of urine, fever, weight loss, concentrated urine, and decrease in skin elasticity. (When your forearm skin is pinched and released, your skin should immediately return to flat.) Increased heart rate, decreased blood pressure, and mental confusion are symptoms in the later stages.

What are the symptoms of decreased sodium (hyponatremia)?

They are non-specific and include poor or no appetite, dizziness, apprehension, decreased blood pressure, nausea, white, pasty color in Caucasians, clammy skin, weakness, decreased reflexes, nausea, abdominal and muscle cramping, headache, swelling, and increase or decrease of the blood pressure.

What does potassium do in the body?

It is used for muscle contraction, sending nerve signals, transforming carbohydrates into energy, and assisting in reassembling amino acids into protein.

What are the symptoms of decreased potassium (hypokalemia)?

They are non-specific and include muscle weakness, abnormal heart rhythm, abdominal distention (enlargement), decreased reflexes, decreased intestinal activity (can lead to gas and constipation, vomiting if severe enough), fatigue, vomiting, increased heart rate, depression, and poor or no appetite. In an extremely severe case, mental confusion and serious irregular heart rhythms can occur.

How does a doctor know for sure if there is dehydration or a problem with sodium, potassium, calcium, and/or magnesium blood levels?

By testing your blood. A "serum electrolyte" test will check on potassium and sodium, and other tests can check on water concentration.

Why can't I just use the caffeine in coffee as my diuretic?

Several reasons: Caffeine is only a weak diuretic, working rapidly and leaving the body quickly. It cannot help regulate fluid and sodium balance for long. Caffeine also causes unwanted effects such as blood vessel constriction in the inner ear, brain stimulation, increased gastric acid secretion, and stimulation of the heart.

References

———. *Drug Information for the Health Care Professional*. Rockville: United States Pharmacopeial Convention, 1990.

———. *Physicians' Desk Reference*. Oradell, N.J.: Medical Economics, 1998.

Griffith, H.W. *Complete Guide to Prescription and Non-Prescription Drugs*. Sixth edition. The Body Press, 1989.

Hardman, J.G., Gilman, A.G., and Limbird, L.E. *Goodman and Gilman's: The Pharmacological Basis of Therapeutics*. Ninth edition. New York: McGraw-Hill, 1996.

Katzung, B.G. *Basic and Clinical Pharmacology*. Sixth edition. Norwalk, Connecticut: Appleton and Lange, 1995.

Long, J.W., and Rybacki, J.J. *The Essential Guide to Prescription Drugs*. New York: Harper Perennial, 1994.

McEvoy, G.K. *AHFS Drug Information*. Bethesda: American Society of Hospital Pharmacists, 1990.

Ruckenstein, M.J., Rutka, J.A., and Hawke, M. "The Treatment of Meniere's Disease: Torok Revisited." *Laryngoscope*, 101:211-218, 1991.

Santos, P.M., Hall, R.A., Snyder, J.M., Hughes, L.F., and Dobie, R.A. "Diuretic and Diet Effect on Meniere's Disease Evaluated by the 1985 Committee on Hearing and Equilibrium Guidelines." *Otolaryngology-Head and Neck Surgery,* 109(4):680-689, 1993.

Scherer, J.C., and Roach, S.S. *Introductory Clinical Pharmacology.* Fifth edition. Philadelphia: Lippincott, 1996.

Silverman, H.M. *The Pill Book.* Seventh edition. New York: Bantam Books, 1996.

Slattery, W.H., and Fayad, J.N. "Medical Treatment of Meniere's Disease." *Otolaryngologic Clinics of North America,* 3(6):1027-1037, 1997.

Wilson, B.A., Shannon, M.T., and Stang, C.L. *Nurses' Drug Guide 1993.* Norwalk: Appleton and Lange, 1993.

Chapter 23

Drugs Meant to Block Symptoms Temporarily

The best treatment is one that eliminates the cause of a problem. Because the underlying cause of Meniere's disease is unknown, it is difficult to attack it directly. When a cure is not available, blocking the symptoms becomes the next goal. Drugs exist that can block symptoms temporarily without permanently changing the vestibular system.

Unfortunately hearing, tinnitus, and ear fullness are not usually helped by these drugs. However, vertigo, nausea, vomiting, and "fight or flight" symptoms can be lessened or blocked successfully in many people.

Symptom-blocking drugs are grouped into three categories in this chapter:

- "Motion sickness" drugs: meclizine (Antivert, etc.), dimenhydrinate (Dramamine, etc.), diphenhydramine (Benadryl, etc.), and scopolamine.
- Drugs used for nausea and vomiting: promethazine (Phenergan), prochlorperazine (Compazine, etc.) and trimethobenzamide (Tigan, etc.).
- Anti-anxiety/anti-vertigo drugs: diazepam (Valium), alprazolam (Xanax), lorazepam (Ativan), and clonazepam (Klonopin).

Although these drugs belong to different groups and work in different ways, there are some similarities, as follows:

- They should not be used with alcohol, barbiturates, tranquilizers, sleeping medicine, allergy medicines, anesthetics, pain medications, sedatives, antidepressants, marijuana or other street drugs, or with each other unless under the direction of a physician. Any drug that causes depression of the brain will also increase their effect and can cause great drowsiness.
- Many of these drugs can cause a dry mouth. For a dry mouth try rinsing your mouth, drinking fluids, sucking on ice or sugar-free hard candy, or taking a saliva substitute such as Moi-Stir, or

Xero-Lube. If you experience a dry mouth much of the time, see your dentist; a dry mouth can increase the likelihood of tooth decay and gum disease.

• Drowsiness is common with many of these drugs. You should not drive or do anything else requiring coordination and thorough thought if you are experiencing drowsiness. Do not drive if your vision is blurry.

• Many of these drugs are antihistamines. If you are taking one of them and are sent for allergy testing, remind your primary doctor that you are taking it since it may interfere with the testing. Also, inform the allergist that you are taking the drug.

• Antihistamines may cause histamine and betahistine to become ineffective; alternatively, histamine and betahistine can interfere with the usefulness of antihistamines.

In this chapter, we have included more information on drugs that are available over-the-counter than on drugs available by prescription only since people taking the over-the-counter variety may not have as much information from other sources. More information about all of the drugs in this chapter (and other drugs sometimes used to treat Meniere's disease) is available from your physician and your pharmacist.

Motion Sickness Drugs

Special note: If you develop eye pain, see halos around lights, or develop blurred vision (all symptoms of glaucoma) while taking any of the motion sickness drugs, report it to your doctor.

Meclizine

Also known as: **Antivert, Bonine, Dizmiss, Antrizine, Meni-D, Ru-vert-M, Motion Cure.** In Canada, **Wehvert** and **Bonamine.**

Meclizine is an over-the-counter antihistamine used to decrease or stop nausea, vomiting, and the dizziness of motion sickness. It acts directly on the inner ear, is able to decrease the amount of vestibular information the brain receives, and acts on the area of the brain responsible for nausea and vomiting. This antihistamine may be effective in some people because it might work on the effects of an inner ear allergy rather than just working on motion sickness.

Meclizine begins to work 30 to 60 minutes after you take it. Its peak of action occurs in one to two hours and continues for eight to 24 hours.

Meclizine can also be obtained with a prescription. Check with your pharmacist to determine the least expensive product you can purchase. A prescription from your doctor may be less expensive than buying an over-the-counter product.

Limits

Not everyone can use meclizine. People with asthma, glaucoma, emphysema, prostate enlargement, heart failure, intestinal blockage, heart rhythm problems, liver disease, urinary tract blockage, pulmonary (lung) disease, someone missing substantial vestibular function in both ears, and/or someone who is pregnant may be told by their doctors not to take this drug.

If you are asked to take this drug regularly, you can expect the drowsiness to decrease, maybe even disappear.

Dimenhydrinate

Also known as: **Dramamine, Dramilin, Calm-X, Marmine, Tega-Vert, Triptone** caplets, and **Travel Aids.** In Canada, **Nauseatol, Novo-Dimenate, Traveltabs,** and **Gravol.**

Dimenhydrinate is an over-the-counter antihistamine used to decrease or stop nausea and vomiting and the dizziness of motion sickness. It begins to work 15 to 30 minutes after you swallow it and lasts four to six hours.

Limits

If you have prostate problems, glaucoma, urinary tract blockage or difficulty urinating, asthma, heart rhythm problems, convulsive disorders, stomach ulcers and/or significant bilateral vestibular losses, you may be told by your doctor not to take dimenhydrinate.

If you are instructed to take this drug on a daily schedule, the drowsiness can be expected to decrease, maybe even disappear.

Diphenhydramine

Also known as: **Benadryl, Belix, Allermax, Beldin, Banophen**.

Diphenhydramine is another over-the-counter antihistamine used to decrease or stop nausea, vomiting, and the dizziness of motion sickness. It begins to work in 60 minutes, hits peak action in two to four hours, and lasts four to seven hours.

Limits

People with acute asthma, glaucoma, stomach ulcer, peptic ulcer, urinary tract obstruction, hyperthyroidism, gastrointestinal (GI) obstruction or stenosis (narrowing), convulsive disorders, cardiovascular disease, diabetes mellitus, thyroid disease, heart disease, asthma, epilepsy and/or pregnant women may be told by their doctors not to take the drug.

If you are instructed to take this drug on a daily schedule, the drowsiness can be expected to decrease, maybe even disappear.

Scopolamine

Also known as: **Transderm-Scop.** In Canada, **Transderm-V.**

Scopolamine, the only drug in this group that is not an antihistamine, is available by prescription to prevent the nausea and vomiting of motion sickness. It usually does not affect the violent vertigo of an attack of Meniere's disease. The patch is designed to deliver medication for three days; the best effects are not available until the patch has been in place for as long as 12 hours.

Cautions

• Do not rub your eyes after applying or removing the scopolamine patch unless you have washed your hands.
• Be careful not to get overheated while taking this drug since it may decrease your ability to sweat. Exercise, hot weather, hot tubs, saunas, etc., may cause you to become lightheaded.

Warning

Most doctors do not prescribe scopolamine for use on a regular basis in Meniere's disease because many people go through a withdrawal period when stopping the drug. Withdrawal symptoms can include dizziness, nausea, vomiting, headache, disturbances of equilibrium, return of vertigo, anxiety, irritability, nightmares, and trouble sleeping. Tolerance to the drug may also occur; that is, the same amount of the drug may no longer bring about the same amount of relief.

Drugs Used for Nausea, Vomiting

The medications most commonly prescribed to prevent or stop nausea and vomiting associated with vestibular symptoms are described in this section.

Promethazine

Also known as: **Phenergan.**

Promethazine is both an antihistamine and phenothiazine derivative available only by prescription. It is used for sedation and to stop nausea and vomiting caused by motion sickness or other factors. It is available for home use as a tablet, oral solution, and as a rectal suppository, and it works within 20 minutes.

Suppositories should be stored in a refrigerator between 36 and 46 degrees Fahrenheit.

Prochlorperazine

Also known as: **Compazine, Stemetil, Chlorazine.**

Prochlorperazine, a prescription medicine, is used for its anti-nausea and anti-vomiting properties. It is not thought to be effective in preventing vertigo or motion sickness. It is available for home use as a tablet, oral solution, extended-release capsule, and rectal suppository. The suppository works within 60 minutes and the tablets/caplets work within 30 to 40 minutes.

This drug can cause side effects called an extrapyramidal reaction.

In depth: Extrapyramidal reactions or symptoms are side effects that can occur when a drug affects certain areas of the brain. Extrapyramidal reactions can be grouped into three types: acute dystonic reactions, akathisia, and Parkinsonism.

Acute dystonic reactions may include neck muscle or back spasms, mandibular tics (jaw jerking), and difficulty talking. These reactions usually occur within 24 to 48 hours of starting drug therapy or when there is an increase in drug dose.

Motor restlessness or akathisia includes agitation, jitteriness, inability to sit still, tapping of the feet, or a strong urge to move around. In most cases akathisia occurs within two to three days of therapy, although it can occur later (up to several weeks).

Parkinsonism appears as a mask-like face, drooling, tremors, pill-rolling motion of the fingers and/or a shuffling gait (walk).

In addition to extrapyramidal reactions, a dyskinesia (tardive dyskinesia) or difficulty in performing voluntary movements can occur. Tardive dyskinesia appears as rhythmic, involuntary movements of the tongue, face, mouth, or jaw. It may occur after long term administration of agents like prochlorperazine, or after a certain cumulative (total) dose is reached.

Trimethobenzamide

Also known as: **Tigan, Arrestin, Tebamide, Ticon, Tigect, T-Gen.**

Trimethobenzamide is another prescription antihistamine that works on the nausea and vomiting center in the brain. Available for home use as a capsule or rectal suppository, it begins to work in 10 to 40 minutes, and its effect lasts three to four hours.

Anti-Anxiety Drugs

The anti-anxiety drugs described in this section are all known as benzodiazepines. They act in the brain to produce their effects. They decrease anxiety, have a calming effect, can suppress vertigo, can cause drowsiness and sleep, can have muscle relaxant and anti-convulsant effects, and can cause amnesia. They are all prescription drugs and have the ability to cause addiction.

None should be stopped abruptly if they have been taken routinely daily for four to six weeks or longer. Withdrawal symptoms can occur when these drugs are stopped abruptly or if the dose is severely reduced. These drugs stay in the body for days after the drug is stopped, so withdrawal symptoms may not occur until a few days later.

Diazepam

Also known as: **Valium, Valcaps, Vazepam.** In Canada: **Novo-Dipam, Vivol.**

Diazepam is used to decrease anxiety, decrease muscle tension, and to cover up vestibular symptoms. Its effects can be felt in 30 minutes.

In depth (withdrawal): Withdrawal symptoms can include tremor, difficulty concentrating, anxiety, agitation, increased sensitivity to light and sound, strange sensations, numbness/tingling, muscle jerking, sleep disturbances, depersonalization, abnormal perception of movement, dizziness, abdominal and muscle cramps, vomiting, sweating, and convulsions.

The symptoms of withdrawal may seem more like a return of the original symptoms than a reaction to stopping the drug.

Alprazolam

Also known as: **Xanax.**

Alprazolam is used to decrease anxiety and to cover up vestibular symptoms. The pill form begins to work within one to two hours.

Special warning: This drug has been confused by some people with the drug Zantac, a stomach medication available by prescription and over-the-counter. Double check your medicine before taking it, particularly if you are taking a large number of drugs.

Avoid drinking grapefruit juice within several hours of taking alprazolam, since the combination may result in significant enhanced effects of the alprazolam. (Enhanced means it will become stronger then intended by the prescribing physician.)

Withdrawal symptoms can include heightened sensory perception, impaired concentration, muscle cramps, decreased appetite, weight loss, muscle twitch, diarrhea, blurred vision, and numbness or a tingling sensation.

When alprazolam is used to treat panic disorder, stopping the drug can cause a "rebound" of the symptoms, a reappearance of panic at or above the level previously experienced.

Lorazepam

Also known as: **Ativan, Alzapam.**
Lorazepam is used to decrease anxiety and vestibular symptoms. Besides being available in tablet form, it is also available as a sublingual tablet that can be placed under the tongue, from where it is absorbed into the blood stream. The peak effect of lorazepam usually occurs in two hours.

Clonazepam

Also known as: **Klonopin, Rivotril.**
Clonazepam is used to decrease vestibular symptoms. It begins to work within one hour with its peak action occurring in one to two hours.

References

_____. *Drug Information for the Health Care Professional.* Rockville: United States Pharmacopeial Convention, 1990.

_____. *Physicians' Desk Reference.* Oradell, N.J.: Medical Economics, 1998.

_____. *The PDR Family Guide to Prescription Drugs.* Montvale, NJ: Medical Economics, 1995.

Baloh, R.W., and Halmagyi, M.G. *Disorders of the Vestibular System.* New York: Oxford University Press, 1996.

Griffith, H.W. *Complete Guide to Prescription and Non-Prescription Drugs.* Sixth edition. The Body Press, 1989.

Hardman, J.G., Gilman, A.G., and Limbird. L.E. *Goodman and Gilman's: The Pharmacological Basis of Therapeutics.* Ninth edition. New York: McGraw-Hill, 1996.

Katzung, B.G. *Basic and Clinical Pharmacology.* Sixth edition. Norwalk, Connecticut: Appleton and Lange, 1995.

Norris, C.H. "Drugs Affecting the Inner Ear: A Review of Their Clinical Efficacy, Mechanisms of Action, Toxicity, and Place in Therapy." *Drugs,* 36:754-772, 1988.

Silverman, H.M. *The Pill Book.* Seventh edition. New York: Bantam Books, 1996.

Slattery, W.H., and Fayad, J.N. "Medical Treatment of Meniere's Disease." *Otolaryngologic Clinics of North America,* 3(6):1027-1037, 1997.

Chapter 24

Steroids

Steroids are hormones your body naturally produces to carry out or to assist in many of its normal activities and during times of stress. Sometimes taking additional steroids (drugs) can help stop an abnormal condition or can mask negative symptoms caused by an abnormal condition. When taken as drugs, steroids are quite potent. The steroids used to treat the inner ear are more properly called "corticosteroids," but we will use the term "steroid" here because more people are familiar with it.

Note: Autoimmune inner ear disease (AIED), one cause of symptoms resembling those of Meniere's disease, can sometimes be successfully treated and stopped by steroids.

How Steroids Work

Steroids are replacement drugs for the adrenal gland. When entering the body, they activate cells that regulate the balance of electrolytes, glucose, lipids, etc., and inhibit inflammatory reaction by decreasing most of the white blood cells. The way steroids work in the ear is not fully understood, but they decrease the number of cells going into an area of infection or inflammation, stop the work of many cells responsible for the body's inflammatory response, and decrease capillary permeability. They may also increase blood flow within the cochlea.

In depth (capillary): A capillary is the smallest blood vessel in the body. It delivers oxygen and nutrients to the body's cells and removes waste products. High permeability refers to a state in which the little opening that lets substances out of the capillary does not close properly and allows more fluid than usual to flow outside. This causes swelling.

In the case of treatment for Meniere's disease, steroids are given in an effort to treat the inflammation that may be present within the inner ear or to stop an immune reaction that may be present.

Some doctors treat all the people first coming to them with the symptoms of Meniere's disease with steroids and perhaps a symptom blocker like meclizine or diazepam (Valium).

Systemic Steroids

Systemic steroids are used for two possible reasons. One is to attack the cause of the Meniere's disease, and the other is to decrease inner ear inflammation no matter what the cause. The cause of Meniere's disease may well be at a distance from the inner ear itself. A systemic drug should reach it in most locations.

When steroids are given systemically, they can cause any of a number of significant changes in many areas of the body. These changes depend upon the amount of drug given at one time, the length of time it was given, how it was given, and which steroid was given. (Some steroids are much stronger than others.)

See Table 24-1 for a list of bodily changes that systemic steroids can cause.

Table 24-1: Bodily Changes that Systemic Steriods Can Cause	
acne	increased susceptibility to
altered mood (euphoria, anger, depression, etc.)	infection
	insomnia
blood pressure changes	increased fragility ("thinning")
bone weakening (including osteoporosis)	of the skin
	increased appetite
bruising	mouth fungus
cataract formation	muscle weakness
decreased potassium levels	menstrual irregularities
glaucoma	nausea
hair growth in abnormal places	obscured signs and symptoms of infection
headache	pancreatitis
heartburn	peptic ulcer
increased sodium levels	redistribution of fat resulting in a
increased blood sugar	full face (sometimes referred to
increased blood cholesterol levels	as a "moon face")
	swelling
increased sensitivity to heat	vomiting
impaired wound healing	weight gain

Reporting to Your Doctor

You should ask your doctor or his or her representative directly what information you should report to them if you are taking systemic steroids. In general, you should report vomiting for more than

12 hours, stomach or abdominal pain, elevated temperature, muscle weakness or cramping, the start of or an increase in blurred vision, cloudy vision, eye pain, bone pain, broken bones, sore throat, and calf pain.

Preventing Problems

To avoid problems with steroids, you should:

- Avoid overheating (sauna, hot tub, midday sun).
- Don't take your steroid drug on an empty stomach.
- If you have a "sensitive" stomach, discuss it with your doctor before problems occur.
- Take care of cuts that occur. Keep them clean and dry.
- If you are on a low-sodium diet, stick to it closely. Even if you are not on a low-sodium diet, avoid salty foods like pickles and potato chips.
- Have eye examinations at least yearly.
- Treat your feet well. Avoid blisters and ingrown nails that could become infected.

The list of significant possible side effects of systemic steroids is big. If you are only on a steroid for a week or two, the chances of developing any serious side effect is less than if you take it for months or years. The side effects are not mentioned here to scare you; they are here to help keep you safe.

Can Everyone Take Systemic Steroids?

Not everyone can take systemic steroids safely. People with a peptic ulcer, tuberculosis (current or old), diabetes mellitus, high blood pressure, thrombophlebitis, myasthenia gravis, deficient thyroid, or an active herpes simplex virus eye infection might be told they should not take steroids systemically.

Warning: Steroids are a category of drugs that should not be stopped or withdrawn abruptly. If you are taking systemic steroids, get and wear a medic alert kind of necklace/bracelet, and carry the information about your drugs in your wallet or purse. Make sure your relatives know you are taking a medicine that should not be stopped suddenly. Sudden withdrawal from a steroid can result in severe sickness, sometimes life-threatening, not only because the body is getting less steroids as medication but because it makes less of its own when receiving "outside" steroids and needs time to resume its normal production.

Tell every health care provider you see, including your dentist, that you are taking systemic steroids. This will enable all of your health care providers to give you the best care for your particular situation.

Steroid withdrawal symptoms can include muscle pain, joint pain (possibly severe), fever, and malaise.

In order to prevent withdrawal symptoms and to allow the adrenal glands (the body's makers of steroids) to recover from drug-induced changes, your doctor will set up a specific schedule for you to follow when you "come off" steroids (sometimes referred to as "tapering" or "weaning"). If you follow the schedule carefully, you should not experience serious withdrawal symptoms.

Local Steroids

Over the last four years, there has been a trend in the U.S. toward placing a steroid into the middle ear in addition to giving it systemically.

The steroid dexamethasone (Decadron) is used in this procedure. The procedure itself might be referred to as transtympanic dexamethasone treatment, transtympanic steroid treatment, intratympanic dexamethasone treatment, or intratympanic steroid treatment. Dexamethasone is a steroid that works for a long time and has the highest anti-inflammatory potency of any steroid. (At least, this is the case when the drug is given systemically; it is too soon to tell if this is also the case with local administration into the ear.)

Through early 1998, little has been published about this procedure in textbooks and scientific journals, but more should become available as studies are completed.

How It's Done

Approaches to this treatment vary from one doctor to the next. Most published reports describe surgically entering the middle ear and placing the dexamethasone near the round window while the person being operated on is under general anesthetic or heavy sedation. At the same time, dexamethasone is also given by IV (intravenously). Dexamethasone in pill form may also be prescribed for up to three months after this surgery.

Potential Complications or Side Effects

Because the procedure is so new, most of the possible problems are theoretical. For example, a report by H. Silverstein and others about a group of people treated with an intratympanic steroid said that none of the people lost hearing; however, the report listed hearing loss as a possible consequence of the procedure because injecting something into the middle ear through the tympanic membrane might cause damage.

Possible complications include:
- hearing loss
- increased tinnitus
- increased aural fullness
- infection
- tympanic membrane perforation
- ear drainage
- unpredictable events
  If general anesthesia is used, its risks must be added to this list.

Concepts to Remember

- Steroids are potent drugs.
- Those given by mouth should not be stopped suddenly.
- Often they are used as symptom-blocking drugs.
- Sometimes they are used to treat causes of problems.
- As of early 1998, transtympanic administration of dexamethasone is new in the U.S. Because it has not been thoroughly tested or reported upon, it is considered by some authorities to be controversial.

References

Griffith, H.W. *Complete Guide to Prescription and Non-Prescription Drugs.* Sixth edition. The Body Press, 1989.

Hardman, J.G., Gilman, A.G., and Limbird, L.E. *Goodman and Gilman's: The Pharmacological Basis of Therapeutics.* Ninth edition. New York: McGraw-Hill, 1996.

Itoh, A., and Sakata, E. "Treatment of Vestibular Disorders." *Acta Otolaryngologica, Supplement,* 481:617-623, 1991.

Nadel, D.M. "The Use of Systemic Steroids in Otolaryngology." *Ear, Nose and Throat Journal,* 75:502-516, 1996.

Scherer, J.C., and Roach, S.S. *Introductory Clinical Pharmacology.* Fifth edition. Philadelphia: Lippincott, 1996.

Shea, J.J., and Ge, X. "Dexamethasone Perfusion of the Labyrinth Plus Intravenous Dexamethasone for Meniere's Disease." *Otolaryngologic Clinics of North America,* 29(2):353-358, 1996.

Shea, J.J., "The Role of Dexamethasone or Streptomycin Perfusion in the Treatment of Meniere's Disease." *Otolaryngologic Clinics of North America,* 30(6):1051-1059, 1997.

Silverman, H.M. *The Pill Book.* Seventh edition. New York: Bantam Books, 1996.

Silverstein, H., Choo, D., Rosenberg, S.I., Kuhn, J., Seidman, M., and Stein, I. "Intratympanic Steroid Treatment of Inner Ear Disease and Tinnitus (Preliminary Report)." *Ear, Nose and Throat Journal,* 75(8):4468-474, 1996.

Wilson, B.A., Shannon, M.T., and Stang, C.L. *Nurses' Drug Guide 1993.* Norwalk: Appleton and Lange, 1993.

Chapter 25

Miscellaneous Drugs

T his chapter reviews drugs that don't fit into any of the other categories in the drug section and are not frequently used in the U.S. For a complete review of side effects, interactions and other facts, ask your physician or pharmacist. You may also want to refer to the reference sections of Chapters 21-26 for books and articles you can read to help you discuss your treatment with your doctor.

Miscellaneous drugs are divided into:
• blood flow drugs
• calcium channel blockers

Blood Flow Drugs

Nicotinic acid (niacin), Betahistine (Serc), and histamine are drugs prescribed by doctors who think that the problem in Meniere's disease could be impaired blood flow to the inner ear. It is thought that blood vessels are enlarged by these drugs and that this allows more blood into the inner ear to help remove excess endolymph. It is hoped that this reduction in endolymph will decrease or stop the vertigo attacks and perhaps the tinnitus, aural fullness/pressure, and hearing loss.

It is difficult to say with any accuracy how commonly these drugs are used, but nicotinic acid and histamine seem to be used much less often now than in the past. The use of betahistine, however, is common in Canada, Mexico, the United Kingdom, and in much of Europe.

Nicotinic Acid or Vitamin B-3

Nicotinic acid is a water-soluble B vitamin available over the counter. Physicians recommending its use do so because of its ability to enlarge blood vessels (in general) and its ability to lower cholesterol levels. Although it is available without a prescription, it has been linked to hepatitis and other problems in some people taking it. As with any other medication, discuss its use with your physician.

Special note: If you take nicotinic acid, take it with meals.

Coping

Nicotinic acid is different from most of the other drugs because of its most notable side effect, flushing, a sudden skin redness and warmth, usually of the face, neck, and chest. If your skin becomes too hot while you're at home, a cool shower may give some relief. A cool, wet cloth to the forehead may be beneficial.

Histamine

Histamine is a chemical normally found throughout the body. It is involved in allergy and inflammatory responses, gastric acid secretion, and acts as a neurotransmitter (sends messages within the nervous system). It produces the kinds of responses antihistamines are used to counter.

This drug can be taken as a drop under the tongue or by injection. The doctors who give histamine intravenously usually do so in the emergency room to treat violent attacks of vertigo.

Histamine is probably ineffective if taken with antihistamines.

Special note: If you are being sent for allergy testing, tell the allergist that you have received histamine and when you had the last dose.

Betahistine (Serc)

Betahistine hydrochloride is only available in the U.S. from a pharmacist who does compounding with a doctor's prescription. Serc, the mass-produced version of betahistine, is not approved for use in the U.S. by the Food and Drug Administration but is available in Canada, Mexico, Great Britain, and throughout most of Europe.

Definition: Compounding is the preparation of a drug from raw products or ingredients. All pharmacists are trained in college to compound, but many do not routinely provide the service.

Some people claim betahistine can prevent attacks of Meniere's disease. However, it is not thought to stop the progression of damage from the disease, and it may not stop tinnitus, aural pressure, or hearing loss.

It is speculated that betahistine may have a vasodilator effect that improves blood flow in the microcirculation of the inner ear. It could also affect vestibular compensation within the brain.

People with bronchial asthma, pheochromocytoma, and/or peptic ulcer (active or in the past) should not take this drug.

Special note: If you are being sent for allergy testing, tell the allergist that you have received betahistine and when you had the last dose.

Betahistine's action may be reduced or prevented by the simultaneous use of antihistamines.

Calcium Channel Blockers; Antihistamines

Two drugs, cinnarizine and flunarizine, are commonly used in Europe to treat Meniere's disease in general and motion sickness symptoms in particular. These drugs are both calcium channel blockers and antihistamines. Drugs that block calcium channels manipulate the way calcium enters body cells. They probably work as symptom blockers.

Cinnarizine has been used in Europe since 1966 and flunarizine since 1985 for motion sickness, to block vertigo, and for Meniere's disease. These drugs are not approved by the Food and Drug Administration for use in the U.S. (However, some doctors prescribe drugs that are simply calcium channel blockers.)

Caution

Do not drive or do anything else requiring coordination and thorough thought if you are experiencing drowsiness from these drugs. Do not drive if your vision is blurry.

Avoid alcohol when taking these drugs.

References

Brookes, G.B. "Meniere's Disease: A Practical Approach to Management." *Drugs*, 25: 77-89, 1983.

Haid, T. "Evaluation of Flunarizine in Patients with Meniere's Disease: Subjective and Vestibular Findings." *Acta Otolaryngologica, Supplement*, 460:149-153, 1988.

Norris, C.H. "Drugs Affecting the Inner Ear: A Review of Their Clinical Efficacy, Mechanisms of Action, Toxicity, and Place in Therapy." *Drugs*, 36:754-772, 1988.

Slattery, W.H., and Fayad, J.N. "Medical Treatment of Meniere's Disease." *Otolaryngologic Clinics of North America,* 3(6):1027-1037, 1997.

Chapter 26

Drugs Meant to Block Symptoms Permanently

B locking vertigo permanently sounds like just the thing everyone with Meniere's disease would want. Unfortunately, it is more complicated than it sounds. The only way to stop symptoms permanently is to stop nearly all vestibular messages, good ones as well as bad, by destroying either the vestibular hair cells or cutting the vestibular nerve.

The drugs used to permanently block vertigo are two aminoglycoside antibiotics, streptomycin and gentamicin. These drugs are not used for their antibiotic properties; they are used because of a side effect, ototoxicity (ear poisoning).

Two different treatments, gentamicin treatment of one ear and streptomycin treatment of both ears, use aminoglycoside antibiotics. These procedures are sometimes referred to generally as chemical destruction or chemical ablation.

Gentamicin Treatment of One Ear

Some other names for the gentamicin treatment are intratympanic gentamicin, transtympanic gentamicin, chemical labyrinthectomy, and pharmacologic labyrinthectomy.

How Does Gentamicin Treatment Work?

The rationale behind any destructive treatment, including this one, is that the brain can adapt to complete loss of balance signals better than fluctuating signals, the problem commonly encountered in Meniere's disease.

This drug destroys vestibular hair cells. Once most of the hair cells of one ear are destroyed, balance signals are no longer sent to the brain from the treated side. When most or all of the faulty signals stop, so do the violent episodes of vertigo (in most people). When the signals stop, the way your brain controls your balance changes forever. This change may or may not be a problem now or later in your life.

In reality, the balance hair cells in a treated ear are usually not all destroyed by gentamicin treatments. This can be good or bad. It's possible that the remaining hair cells will help you maintain balance better than expected. It's also possible that the remaining cells will continue to cause problems either now or in the future.

When Do Doctors Offer Gentamicin Treatment?

Gentamicin treatment is usually offered to someone who has Meniere's disease in one ear, who doesn't improve with medical treatment including low-sodium diet, diuretics, and temporary symptom blockers, and who is disabled by the symptoms. In the U.S., this treatment has been offered only for the last six or so years. Not all doctors offer this option to their patients.

How Is Gentamicin Put in One Ear?

Gentamicin is placed into the middle ear and enters the inner ear through the round window and the oval window. Placement is accomplished in one of the following ways:
• Gentamicin is injected through the tympanic membrane during each treatment.
• A micro-catheter is inserted through the tympanic membrane and left in place during the treatments.
• A surgery is done to lift the tympanic membrane and place gentamicin directly on the round window.

If the gentamicin is placed into the middle ear, the head is positioned to prevent the fluid from rolling down the eustachian tube and to maximize the gentamicin's contact with the oval and round windows. This head position may be maintained for 60 minutes or longer.

The amount of gentamicin and the timing of treatments varies quite a bit from one doctor to the next. The number of treatments needed varies from person to person. It is generally thought that giving the treatments at widely-spaced intervals rather than over successive days reduces the chance of hearing loss dramatically.

How Will I Maintain My Balance?

Each inner ear sends balance information to the vestibular nuclei. The left inner ear sends its information to the left vestibular nuclei and the right ear to the right vestibular nuclei. When one ear is treated with gentamicin, many of its balance signals stop arriving at its vestibular nuclei. After a period of adjustment, the brain can make balance decisions based mainly on information from the good ear. This change in the vestibular nuclei is referred to as *compensation*.

Does Everybody Compensate?

Not everybody compensates. If your brain can't make this adjustment, you may have symptoms similar to those felt for a couple of days after a big attack of Meniere's disease: unsteadiness, difficulty when turning your head rapidly, fogginess, etc.

Who Will Be Unable to Compensate?

Older people usually have a greater problem with compensation. Someone whose balance problem is located in the brain rather than the ear will probably not be able to compensate. And if the opposite ear also has Meniere's disease, compensation may be hindered.

Can Compensation Be Undone?

Compensation might be reversed. Some drugs and alcohol can cause temporary "decompensation" as can some illnesses and fatigue. Meniere's disease in the other ear can also undo compensation.

What About Hearing?

When gentamicin is given, it enters the inner ear through the cochlea before entering the vestibular areas. Therefore, the possibility of damage to hearing hair cells exists. When the gentamicin treatment is given on consecutive days, there is a 25 to 69 percent chance or greater that some hearing will be lost. When it is given once a week or once every two weeks, the danger to hearing lessens considerably but still might be as high as 25 to 33 percent.

Your doctor will perform hearing tests during your weeks of treatment to monitor your hearing.

Is Being Deaf in One Ear a Big Deal?

Both ears are needed to determine the direction sound is coming from. If you are deaf in one ear and are looking for someone who yells, "I'm over here," you won't be able to determine what direction this call is coming from unless you can see who is yelling. It will also be difficult to follow a conversation in a noisy environment such as a restaurant, to follow a conversation in a car, or to hear sounds in your immediate environment when you are on the phone.

Can Gentamicin Affect My Good Ear?

Because your inner ear is served by blood vessels, it's possible that a small amount of the drug may make it into the blood stream. However, even if the entire amount of drug placed into the ear got into the blood stream, it is unlikely it could cause a problem in the opposite ear.

What Is the Success Rate?

Success is usually defined by the absence of discrete attacks of vertigo. Most studies describe vertigo attacks stopping in 65 to 95 percent of all cases after one series of treatments and 90 percent or better after re-treatment to those not helped or who relapse after the first round.

What if It Doesn't Work?

If the gentamicin treatment fails, several options remain, including doing nothing, giving more gentamicin, trying more temporary symptom blockers, or trying surgery. The damage of gentamicin is cumulative; if the first series of treatments doesn't work, additional doses can increase the total amount of deliberate damage.

What if the Second Ear Becomes Involved?

It is commonly felt that the symptoms of Meniere's disease in a second ear are milder than those in the first ear. However, if the balance function of your second ear is significantly reduced, your situation will be similar to that described below under streptomycin therapy.

Advantages

The gentamicin treatment may not require general anesthesia, requires only a short recuperation period, and costs less than vestibular nerve section.

Drawbacks

The destruction caused by the gentamicin treatment can't

be reversed; a large number of people (as many as 65 percent in one study) suffer some loss of hearing with this procedure, and some people have suffered total loss of hearing in the treated ear. In addition, the procedure must be repeated in a number of people.

Can I Feel Normal After Gentamicin?

Yes, some people get rid of the attacks of vertigo and return to everything they used to do like driving, riding a bicycle, swimming, and socializing.

Others obtain relief from the attacks of vertigo, but their compensation is not complete enough for things to be exactly the way they were before the sickness started.

This treatment is not an all-or-nothing proposition. Some people get rid of the vertigo attacks but don't get back to what they would call "normal;" others do. Others only get rid of a percentage of the vertigo attacks, and some have no change at all. Some may even feel worse.

Streptomycin Treatment of Both Ears

Some other names for the streptomycin treatment of both ears are titration streptomycin and systemic streptomycin.

How Does Streptomycin Treatment Work?

The rationale behind this treatment is that the brain adjusts to signal loss more readily than to fluctuating signals.

When Do Doctors Use This Treatment?

A few doctors offer streptomycin treatments to someone who has Meniere's disease in both ears, who does not respond to routine medical treatment including low-sodium diet, diuretics, and temporary symptom blockers, and who is experiencing disabling attacks of vertigo. This treatment is used only when all hopes of a spontaneous remission have evaporated and the prospect of a permanent balance disability would be an improvement over the attacks.

How Does Streptomycin Get into Both Ears?

Streptomycin therapy is a systemic treatment because it is injected into a large muscle over days to weeks and is absorbed into the blood stream. It travels throughout the body, including both inner ears.

How Will I Maintain My Balance?

When both ears are treated, fewer inner-ear signals arrive at both vestibular nuclei. Because both sides are receiving less information, compensation, as described above, may not take place. Instead, substitution takes place; you come to rely solely on two kinds of input (visual and proprioceptive) to maintain balance rather than the usual three (visual, proprioceptive, and vestibular).

As your brain adjusts to this change, you may feel as though you are staggering or uncoordinated; you may stand with your feet wider apart than normal and have symptoms when moving your head rapidly. Even after your brain adjusts, you may not be able to walk when your vision is absent; that is, when you are in complete darkness or have your eyes closed. You may have difficulty in dim lighting conditions and on uneven ground. Bouncing vision (oscillopsia) during head movements occurs in some people and can be a problem, and a feeling of imbalance or lack of coordination may persist and possibly be permanent.

Vestibular rehabilitation or physical therapy can be helpful during this adjustment time that could last months, maybe even a year or two.

What About Hearing?

The chance is small that hearing loss will occur when streptomycin is injected into a muscle. As a precaution, your doctor may monitor your hearing periodically during your course of treatment. You should tell your doctor immediately if you experience an increase or other change in tinnitus or a decrease in hearing.

Advantages

This treatment is not a surgery; thus, the usual risks of surgery are avoided. Also, the chance of hearing damage is low, and the procedure rids most people with Meniere's disease of their discrete attacks of disabling vertigo.

Drawbacks

The streptomycin treatment is destructive and irreversible. It leaves people with a permanent disability. The amount of drug needed is unknown and must be determined by rotational testing during the treatment. Even with appropriate testing, the eventual effect of the drug upon someone cannot be predicted. Too little destruction or too much can easily occur. Time is needed for you to recuperate and to learn substitution—the use of vision and proprioception alone to maintain balance. Sometimes more treatment is required later.

What if It Does Not Work?

If streptomycin treatment does not work, the options are to do nothing further or to give more streptomycin. The gentamicin treatment might also be tried.

References

Graham, M. "Bilateral Meniere's Disease: Treatment with Intramuscular Titration Streptomycin Sulfate." *Otolaryngologic Clinics of North America*, 30(6):1097-1100, 1997.

Hellstrom, S., and Odkvist, L. "Pharmacologic Labyrinthectomy." *Otolaryngology Clinics of North America*, 27(2):307-315, 1994.

Hirsch, B.E., and Kamerer, D.B. "Role of Chemical Labyrinthectomy in the Treatment of Meniere's Disease." *Otolaryngologic Clinics of North America*, 30(6):1039-1049, 1997.

Hoffer, M.E., Balough, B., Henderson, J., DeCicco, M., Webster, D., O'Leary, M.J., and Kopke, R. "Use of Sustained Release Vehicles in the Treatment of Meniere's Disease." *Otolaryngologic Clinics of North America*, 30(6):1159-1166, 1997.

LaRouere, M.J., Zappia, J.J., and Graham, M.D. "Titration Streptomycin Therapy in Meniere's Disease: Current Concepts." *American Journal of Otology,* 14(5):474-477, 1993.

Monsell, E.M., Cass, S.P., and Ryback, L.P. "Therapeutic Use of Aminoglycosides in Meniere's Disease." *Otolaryngologic Clinics of North America*, 26(5):737-746, 1993.

Chapter 27

Treatment for Cochlear Problems

Tinnitus

For the majority of people, tinnitus is most annoying during the weeks after it first appears. With time, it blends into the background for many people; it is always present but causes no problems. Even so, a significant number of people find tinnitus to be a big problem.

If you find it hard to concentrate, to follow conversations, and/or if you are kept awake by tinnitus at night, you might benefit from help. One thing you can try on your own to make the sleeping hours more bearable is to play radio static or run a fan while you are trying to sleep. That probably sounds bizarre, but it helps a great many people. It even has a term to describe it, *masking*.

Hearing aid companies make instruments that are worn like and look like hearing aids but which don't amplify sounds from the environment. They make a sound like static that is sent into the ear constantly. These instruments are called tinnitus maskers. They are not really helpful for sleep, but if tinnitus bothers you during the day, a masker might help.

In addition, some drugs have been reported to be of value in the treatment of tinnitus. However, none of them can stop tinnitus in all or even most people.

If you have been to an otologist or otolaryngologist, you have probably met and been tested by an audiologist. To find out more about tinnitus treatments, talk to your audiologist.

Researchers continue to seek ways to relieve tinnitus. For example, the use of gingko biloba to reduce tinnitus is being studied at the House Ear Institute in Los Angeles, and in the United Kingdom a study is underway to test the effectiveness of a device called "Therapak."

To learn about strategies to avoid developing more tinnitus, see Chapter 34, "Preservation, Protection."

If tinnitus is one of your big concerns, you might want to seek information from the American Tinnitus Association. (See Chapter 39, "Where to Get More Information.")

Aural Fullness

For most people with Meniere's disease, aural fullness is only an occasionally annoying symptom. For others, it can be a constant presence and might be painful.

Only three treatments are thought capable of alleviating or stopping this symptom: a low-sodium diet, use of diuretics and, sometimes, a surgical procedure called endolymphatic sac drainage or shunting. (See Chapter 29, "Surgery.")

Aural fullness can disappear at any in time in the course of Meniere's disease and usually decreases in severity in "late" Meniere's disease.

Hearing Loss

Sometimes the hearing loss of Meniere's disease stops progressing on its own, and at other times it seems to stop in response to a low-sodium diet and/or the use of a diuretic. No surgery has been shown to stop hearing loss or bring back the lost hearing of Meniere's disease.

People with hearing loss from Meniere's disease can usually benefit from amplification with hearing aids. Hearing aid technology has not only led to smaller, almost invisible hearing aids, it has produced instruments better able to capture and amplify sounds in only the needed frequencies. To learn more about more about these instruments, speak to the audiologist who works with your ear doctor.

A type of hearing aid called a CROS (contralateral routing of sound) can help someone with one deaf ear and one normal ear (or one ear able to benefit from amplification). If you use this device, you will wear something resembling a hearing aid on both ears. The device on the deaf ear contains a sound receiver and transmitter; it receives sound and transmits it to the device on the other ear. Therefore, if you are deaf on the left side and wearing a CROS, you can hear someone whispering into your left ear.

If you have profound hearing losses in both ears, you might benefit from a cochlear implant. This technology is different from hearing amplification in several ways, as follows:

- It is surgically installed or implanted.
- Only one ear is used, not two.
- Using it to its fullest requires a great deal of therapy.
- A cochlear implant system includes many more parts than a hearing aid. The parts of a cochlear implant system include:

- a catheter with a number of electrodes. The catheter is threaded into the cochlea.
- the cochlear implant. (This is not visible once implanted.)
- a transmitter coil (This is a small circular structure containing a small magnet. The circular structure holds the magnet on your head right over the magnet of the cochlear implant. This enables the transmitter to send signals directly into the receiver/stimulator.)
- the coil's connected magnet
- a receiver/stimulator
- a speech processor (It's the size of a pocket calculator and weights 3.5 oz.)
- a cable
- a microphone (It hangs on the external ear like a behind-the-ear hearing aid.)

Figure 27-1 shows the external parts of a cochlear implant system.

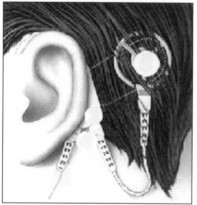

Figure 27-1: External parts of a cochlear implant system.
(Photo courtesy of Cochlear Corporation.)

Hearing with a cochlear implant is not like normal hearing, and the implant is designed to deal with speech not music. Only about half of all cochlear implant users can understand speech without lip reading. Even so, the implant usually improves the user's communication skills. Implants help many people achieve a higher quality of life than was previously possible.

If you want information about hearing aids, cochlear implants, devices for the hearing impaired, or tinnitus maskers, talk to an audiologist. Your otologist or otolaryngologist will have information about these devices but will not usually have had the same thorough training in this area as an audiologist.

For ideas and tips to preserve your remaining hearing, see Chapter 34, "Preservation, Protection."

Chapter 28
Alternative Treatments

The term "alternative treatment" is used in the U.S. to refer to a treatment not used by the majority of medical doctors (also referred to as allopathic doctors) and usually not covered by medical insurance. Alternative treatment is also sometimes referred to as complementary medicine or treatment.

Of course, a treatment like acupuncture may be considered an alternative in the U.S. at the same time it is routine and traditional in China, and though the use of homeopathy is limited in the U.S., members of the British royal family are ministered to by a homeopath. The examples could go on.

Other than being considered alternatives, many of these treatments don't have much in common. Some are aimed at a specific symptom, while others constitute an entire system for staying healthy. Many are aimed at decreasing stress and increasing relaxation. Some of the practitioners of these therapies focus on working in partnership with patients on the mental and emotional aspects of health as well as the physical. It has been suggested that these partnerships themselves may promote health.

In this book, alternative treatments are divided into several categories including those said to work at a distance, those that use some type of bone or muscle manipulation, those that are aimed at mood or the mind, those that use herbs or other medicinals, those that involve movement, those that involve special equipment, and those (miscellaneous) that don't fit neatly into any of these categories. When available, comments by people with Meniere's disease about these treatments have been included.

The interest in alternative treatment is big enough that the National Institutes of Health in Bethesda, Md., has an office for alternative medicine that awards grants (money that is not paid back) for research about such treatments for a great variety of problems. The 1997 budget for this office was $7.4 million. (The total NIH budget was $11.9 billion.)

> **Note:** Don't assume that these treatments can't harm you because they are more "natural." Just because you bought an herbal tea in a health food store does not mean it can't be harmful like a prescription drug. View all substances placed into or onto the body for the purpose of causing a change as a medicine. If you would not take a prescription medication without knowing its side effects, interactions, etc., don't take an herb or other "natural" product without knowing the same things.

Many non-alternative medicines, both over-the-counter and prescription, are also natural. Aspirin comes from the bark of a tree, as does the quinine used to treat malaria, leg cramps, and certain heart rhythm irregularities. Both these drugs are natural and are capable of causing many problems including increased tinnitus. One of the most commonly used heart drugs, digitalis, is made from a beautiful flower, the purple foxglove, and too much of this drug kills just as surely as a poisonous mushroom.

A certain amount of skepticism is natural and probably a good thing. Exercise it with all treatments, not just with some.

VEDA and the author are not endorsing the use of alternative treatments in general or of any specific treatment. Your treatment decisions should be made after complete discussions with your health care provider and after you have learned the risks and benefits of any treatment and discussed these with your spouse or anyone else with whom you usually discuss major decisions.

Treatments Meant to Work at a Distance from the Ear

Acupuncture

Acupuncture is said to be a system for treating the whole person and bringing Yin and Yang back into balance within the body. (In ancient Chinese thought, Yin and Yang are two complementary and opposing forces underlying and controlling all nature.) If you have acupuncture treatment, the acupuncturist will ask questions about your current symptoms and your history. She or he will examine you; usually this will include observation of your skin color and palpation (examination by touch or feeling).

Rebalancing of Yin and Yang is attempted by inserting acupuncture needles into areas around the body (sometimes at a great distance from the area with a problem) for a short time. On occasion, a small electric current may be passed through the needles.

Acupuncture is one of the few alternative treatments that has been studied in relation to Meniere's disease. Two Yugoslavian doctors reported on the subject in the *American Journal of Chinese Medicine*. Their report described 34 people with Meniere's disease who were treated with acupuncture between 1977 and 1981. Vertigo disappeared in all 34 by the third course of treatment, they said, and hearing improved in nearly all cases.

Acupressure

Acupressure treatment is based on the same principles as acupuncture, but instead of inserting needles into various points, the provider applies pressure. The pressure can be applied with the fingertip, knuckle, or an instrument called a *tei shin*.

Reflexology

The providers of reflexology therapy say that the soles of the feet and palms of the hands contain reflex points, also known as areas or zones, that represent all the glands and organs of the body. The application of steady even pressure on the appropriate reflex point is meant to alleviate symptoms.

> "Accidently I discovered that by massaging certain parts of my feet, I could improve my hearing."
> —Anonymous, *Meniere's Disease*
> (Meniere's Australia), 1991.

Body Manipulation

Chiropractic

The basic philosophy of chiropractic says that good health requires that nerve impulses flow unimpeded from the brain down the spinal cord and to all bodily areas. If any bones are out of alignment, they must be returned or adjusted to the proper position by manipulation (placement by hand). Assessment includes physical examination and X-rays. Treatments can include manual adjustments, massage, ultrasound, and heat.

> "A chiropractor did help with my neck aches. . . ."
> - S.T., *Spin 17*, Spring 1996

Craniosacral Therapy

Craniosacral therapy is based on the idea that the brain, spinal column, and sacrum have a continuous column of fluid that can be disturbed by misalignment of the skull, neck, and back bones. A therapist assesses you by feeling along your head, neck, and back for any abnormalities. Treatment is said to attempt to bring everything back into normal alignment.

Rolfing

The stated goal of this treatment is to keep your myofascial system (muscles and connective tissue) properly aligned vertically. Treatment is done using fingers, open hands, fists, and elbows.

Mood/Mind Exercises

Autogenic Training or Autogenics

Autogenic training is said to help focus the power of the mind on relaxation and to try to switch off the fight-or-flight response felt so strongly during attacks of vertigo. This technique has been used by NASA to help the astronauts adapt to space travel.

> "Having tried different relaxation techniques to reduce stress, stiffness in neck and shoulders, and to control the panic at the onset of an attack, I have found autogenic training the most helpful. Autogenic training is based on the principles of meditation, but one does not need superhuman ability to concentrate. It addresses physical and emotional stress in an accessible way. Benefits I experience are greater confidence in managing attacks, more energy to practice my profession and for leisure after working hours, and more calmness in my life."
>
> —D.W., *Spin*, June 1995

Transcendental Meditation

The discipline of transcendental meditation teaches the user to concentrate entirely on a word, called the *mantra*, which is repeated over and over again in the mind. Focus on the mantra diverts the mind from all other thoughts, "the monkeys of the mind." The goal is to produce a state of inner harmony and calm.

> "Regular relaxation and deep breathing can be helpful, and I have learned to meditate."
>
> —E.F., *Spin*, Spring 1996

Imagery, Creative Imagery or Visualization

Instead of taking your mind away from the troubles of your body, visualization therapy teaches you to send positive thoughts, images, or symbols from your mind to your body to help in healing. The process may release endorphins in your brain and lead to pain relief or a general feeling of well-being.

Hypnotherapy

Hypnosis is sometimes used in an attempt to cure a problem or overcome negative symptoms.

Music Therapy

Music therapy uses music in an effort to clear the mind of worries.

Spiritual Healing

Spiritual healing depends upon religion and religious belief to overcome a problem or effect a cure for a disease or disability.

Medicines/Herbs; Other Medicinals

Evening Primrose Oil

Evening primrose oil contains gamma-linoleic acid, which may increase the production of prostaglandins, body substances that might lead to a decrease in inflammation.

> "... and by taking herbal remedies and evening primrose oil, I can, if not eradicate, certainly control it [Meniere's disease] to a point where it does not affect my life."
> —S.Y., *Spin*, June 1995

Gingko Biloba

Gingko biloba is sometimes said to improve tinnitus in some people with inner ear problems. A study is under way at the House Ear Institute in Los Angeles to test this idea.

Herbal Medicine

Herbal medicine uses herbs to maintain health or treat problems.

Homeopathy

Homeopathy involves medicinal use based on the theory that "like cures like." Practitioners of this treatment are trained in a homeopathic college in the use of a multitude of herbs, chemicals, and drugs such as belladonna, borax, wild licorice, and wild hops. These substances are said to stimulate the body's defenses and healing processes.

Ginger Root

Ginger has long been used to decrease the nausea of morning sickness, motion sickness, and other ailments. It can be taken as ginger tea, ginger capsules, ginger snaps, or ginger ale.

Vitamin Therapy

Vitamin therapy refers to the use of vitamins to prevent problems and/or effect a cure. Niacin, vitamin B-3, and lipoflavinoids have been recommended for Meniere's disease by some MDs for years. Like other alternative treatments, vitamin therapy has sometimes produced good results, sometimes mediocre results, sometimes no results, and sometimes bad results.

A zinc deficiency may be a cause of tinnitus in a small percentage of people. Taking zinc may help them. B-12 has also been used by some people to help tinnitus.

Aromatherapy

Aromatherapy involves the use of essential oils made from the flowers, fruits, stems, leaves, or roots of a tree or plant to treat symptoms. The aromatic substances may be massaged into the skin, placed on your bed or your clothing, or directly inhaled. The scent of lavender that has been placed on a pillow case is said to help make people sleepy and ready for sleep. The scent or chemical can enter the body via the nose or through the skin.

If this treatment sounds a bit odd, think about the effect (nausea, vomiting) a bad smell can have on you. Or think of the stimulation that smelling salts can produce. Could a positive smell bring on something good or get rid of something negative?

One "recipe" to relieve stress is to mix five drops of grapefruit oil, four drops of cypress, and two drops of geranium with one teaspoon of vegetable oil. Inhale the aroma, or massage the face, neck, shoulders, chest, and back.

Bach Flower Remedy

The Bach flower treatment is a medicinal therapy with 38 different flower remedies and one combination remedy (called a rescue remedy) mixed into unflavored brandy. The "remedy" is placed under the tongue. The combination remedy is said to be for the instant relief of stress.

Movement

T'ai Chi

T'ai chi is a regimen of exercises practiced widely in China. It consists of slow rhythmic movement from one specific total body position to another done simultaneously with regulated breathing (breathing out slowly, etc.). These positions are specific. Each limb is held in a precise way for a specific length of time. The concept is to do this regimen regularly to help body and "soul" stay in a kind of balance. It is said to clear the mind and relax the body.

If you have a balance impairment, it will usually be more pronounced if you try to stay still or move slowly. T'ai chi forces you to hold a position or move very slowly, and this may give you work on movement where you need it most.

"I have enjoyed T'ai chi, which is calming and helps with balance."

—E.F., *Spin*, Spring 1996.

T'ai chi has not been studied specifically in people with Meniere's disease, but it has been studied in people with poor balance caused by vestibular problems. It was found that after just eight weeks, balance abilities improved enough to be measurable.

Feldenkrais Method

Feldenkrais therapy is based on the theory that usually we learn only enough to get by. To enhance and program the mind and body, we should learn and practice a multitude of exercises or movements, the theory says, so that we may flourish.

Special Equipment

Therapak II

The British manufacturer of the electronic device, Therapak II, claims it is useful in treating the tinnitus and vertigo of Meniere's disease. According to the manufacturer, "The Therapak develops broadband electromagnetic monophasic pulses of a complex wave form and is positioned over the ear typically 15 minutes then 10 minutes behind the neck during treatment."

Ear Candling

Ear candling is an alternative treatment said by its proponents to be helpful for removing ear wax, relieving allergies, and reducing tinnitus. A special candle is inserted into the external auditory canal, and the protruding end is lit. It is said that a gentle vacuum is produced that removes "impurities" from the ear.

Possible complications include external ear burns, occlusion of the external auditory canal with candle wax, a hole through the tympanic membrane, and infection. This list of complications is compiled from those found in a regional survey of otolaryngologists and presented in a letter to the editor of *Archives of Otolaryngology— Head and Neck Surgery.*

Biofeedback

Biofeedback is offered by MDs, physical therapists, and others to help people learn to control body functions not usually under conscious control such as blood pressure, heart rate, digestion, and perspiration. Biofeedback can be used as a treatment for stress and related physical changes.

Whole Person Alternatives

Naturopathy

Naturopathy is a system of health promotion meant to take into account the physical, mental, and spiritual aspects of the individual. These three components are assessed when ill health is present and treatment (chemical, mechanical, or emotional) is given. Naturopathic treatment can take the form of nutrition, herbs, homeopathic medicines, vitamins, massage, and/or Bach flower remedies.

Yoga

"Yoga helps me to relax. Things don't get me down quite as much. I am now able to get on with my life."
—Anonymous, *Meniere's Disease*
(Meniere's Australia), 1991.

Yoga is not just an exercise regimen: it is a system for physical, mental, and spiritual well-being. It includes exercise postures, breathing control, meditation, relaxation, and nutrition.

Miscellaneous

Therapeutic Touch

Therapeutic touch therapy is based on the theory that the body is surrounded by energy that needs to flow unimpeded to maintain good health. Practitioners of therapeutic touch assess the condition of this energy field by placing their hands close to but not in contact with the skin of clients. They claim to use their hands to smooth out problem areas.

Massage

Many types of massage are used to relieve muscle aches, pain, or stiffness, and massage may help to relieve stress. Serotonin may be released by massage, and this may be of benefit to someone with anxiety, depression, or chronic pain.

Massage is a treatment also used by physical therapists in a "traditional" setting.

Hyperbaric Treatment

Hyperbaric treatment exposes someone to oxygen at a pressure greater than the usual pressure of the atmosphere at sea level. More oxygen enters the body and is available for use by the cells.

Hyperbaric treatment is not just alternative medicine; it is also used in "traditional" medicine in situations requiring more oxygen to be delivered to the body. Under certain circumstances, it is also used by divers to prevent the "bends."

Environmental Medicine

Practitioners of environmental medicine look into possible environmental causes of ill-health rather than examining an individual person or his or her mind for a cause. An attempt is made to seek out any cause and effect relationship between something in the environment and someone's symptoms. If a relationship is uncovered or suspected, guidance is given about how to avoid the problem substance. This resembles the idea behind a diet meant to eliminate foods that might be causing allergy problems.

Stress Relief

"I also find stress aggravates any condition, and being a born worrier I have suffered over the years."

—S.Y., *Spin*, June 1995

"The more I worried about having attacks, the more I had, sometimes three a week. . . ."

—E.M.D., *Spin*, June 1995

Comments like these are common among people with Meniere's disease. Preventing or relieving inappropriate stress can only improve the quality of life. Any treatment that can result in a relaxation response is thought to relieve stress.

Getting More Information

How do you go about exploring these "alternative medicine" therapies? Start with your usual health care provider. Some MDs use alternative methods themselves or can refer you to someone who does. Ask your friends, neighbors and relatives if they have any experience with different therapies and the people providing them. Beyond these resources, you can also research the topic at your local library; it will have books and probably current magazines on the topic. Another possible resource is your local health food store. It may carry books and magazines on the topic, and the staff can probably tell you the names of local practitioners of many different types of alternative therapy.

HMOs

If the trend toward using HMOs and other "managed care" arrangements continue, we may see more use or experimentation with alternative therapies in an effort to cut costs. Some HMOs already cover chiropractic care; others are probably not far behind.

References

_____. "CIGNA Health Care for Seniors Guide to Healthy Living." *More Life*, 4(2):4, 1997.

_____. United Kingdom Meniere's Society. *Spin*. June 1995, Spring 1996.

Barton, V. *Meniere's Disease*. Moonah, Tasmania: Meniere's Australia, 1991.

Castelman, M. *Nature's Cures.* Emmaus, Pa.: Rodale Press, Inc., 1996.

Griffin, F.B. "Lipoflavinoids in Meniere's Disease." *Eye, Ear Nose and Throat Monthly,* 49(6):290-291, June 1970.

Hain, Timothy C. "T'ai Chi for Balance Study." http://hsinfo. ghsl.nwu.edu/neuro/programs/vestib/research/taichi.html, June 3, 1997.

Kastner, M., and Burroughs, H. *Alternative Healing: The Complete A-Z Guide to More Than 150 Alternative Therapies:* New York: Henry Holt and Company, 1996.

McElroy, C.E. "Why Alternative Medicine Is Coming Out of the Closet." *Vital Signs,* VII(13):6-7, 1997.

Pfaltz, C.R. *Controversial Aspects of Meniere's Disease.* New York: Thieme, Inc., 1986.

Roland, N.J., *et al.,* "Electromagnetic Stimulation as a Treatment of Tinnitus: A Pilot Study." *Clinical Otolaryngology,* 18:278-281, 1993.

Seely, D.R., and Langman, A.W. "Ear Candles." *Archives of Otolaryngology Head and Neck Surgery,* 121:1068, 1995.

Steinberger, A., and Pansini, M. "The Treatment of Meniere's Disease by Acupuncture." *American Journal of Chinese Medicine,* XI(1-4):102-105, 1983.

Yardley, L. *Vertigo and Dizziness.* London: Routledge, 1994.

Chapter 29
Surgery

As mentioned earlier, the majority of people with Meniere's disease will never have inner ear surgery. They will either improve on their own or while undergoing one medical (non-surgical) treatment or another. The following information may be helpful if you find yourself in the minority who may need to consider surgery.

Treatment Priorities

Surgery is usually not the first choice for treating Meniere's disease because:

• Surgery causes permanent changes.

• It carries risks attached to cutting in or near the ear and to receiving general anesthesia.

• Surgery for any vertigo problem is not a sure thing. It may do nothing, do a little, do a lot, or worsen things.

• Surgery does not guarantee that you will either get better or that you will stay the same. The surgery may provide partial resolution of the symptoms. It may also make existing symptoms and problems worse, or it may create new problems.

• Many surgeries for Meniere's disease work by destroying the vestibular areas of the inner ear or by cutting the nerve sending information to the brain. This permanently changes the way the body's balance mechanisms work, and this change may or may not be a problem in later life, when other changes occur.

• The effectiveness of endolymphatic sac surgeries is controversial. Some studies suggest it is no better over time than doing nothing.

• Surgery is expensive. It costs a great deal more than doing nothing or trying a medical (non-surgical) treatment.

• Although it may block episodic vertigo messages from reaching the brain, surgery does not cure Meniere's disease and stop all the other symptoms. (This same criticism applies to other treatments as well.)

Factors Your Doctor Considers

Physicians look at a number of different factors to determine the best treatment options to offer. These factors or considerations can be divided into three groups: patient, physician, and general.

Patient Factors

- the symptoms, their frequency and severity
- test results
- degree of impairment
- the amount of misery present
- the involvement of one or both ears
- age
- general condition

Physician Factors

- what the doctor was taught in school and during residency training
- what his or her experiences with different treatments have been
- which treatments the doctor believes in or feels have been proven through research
- the doctor's skills and abilities

General Factors

- the risk/benefit ratio
- the availability of facilities

Note on risk/benefit ratio: When determining the appropriateness of a treatment, you and your doctor examine the risks and the possible benefits. The chance of bad results and their severity must be weighed against the chance of positive results and their degree of benefit. A judgment based on this comparison comes down to one question, "Is the possible benefit worth exposure to the risks?"

Questions for Your Doctor

Take the time to ask questions of your doctor, such as:

- What are the alternatives to this surgery? (Make it clear that you want to know about all the alternatives available, not just those offered by your particular doctor or covered by your health insurance plan.)
- Have all the non-invasive treatments been offered and tried?

• What are the risks of the surgery to your general health and to your inner ear (hearing and balance) and nearby anatomic structures?

• What is the best result you could possibly get from surgery? Specifically, how much could the surgery reduce the number or severity of vertigo attacks, the sensations of ear fullness, and the tinnitus, and how much could it improve hearing?

• What is the average or usual result of the surgery?

• What is the worst result that can occur from the surgery?

• How many surgeries like this has your doctor done, and how many resulted in complications?

• When asking about surgical results, try to pin your doctor down on his or her statistics, not those published in the literature by someone else. This someone else might have different skills, different experiences, or access to more sophisticated testing/surgical equipment.

• Doctors use terms like "control of vertigo" or "improvement" when talking about the positive results of surgery and "rare" or "unlikely" when referring to the chance of complications. Do not assume you understand what the doctors mean by these terms unless they actually define them. Ask for their definitions. For example, a doctor in one conversation may say that Meniere's disease is "fairly common" and in another conversation say that a dead ear from endolymphatic sac drainage surgery is "rare." Yet the chance of developing Meniere's disease is about 1 in 500, while the chance of causing a dead ear during sac drainage is between 1 in 50 and 1 in 20.

• Ask your doctor for the names of some people on whom he or she has performed the surgery.

• Ask questions and make sure you understand the answers before deciding about surgery.

Deciding About Surgery

You can make an informed decision about surgery by listening carefully to your doctor, asking questions like the ones above, possibly discussing this information with a trusted friend or relative, and thinking through all options and ramifications of the proposed procedure.

Get a second opinion. There are many schools of thought about the treatment of Meniere's disease. On occasion a physician can become overly enthusiastic about a surgical procedure. For example:

"The cure of Meniere's disease by section of the auditory nerve intracranially is now established. Following this operative procedure, which has now been employed in 35 cases, there have been no subsequent attacks of dizziness, no loss of life, and no disturbance of function, except in two of the early cases when the facial nerve was injured—a danger which is now scarcely possible."

—W.E. Dandy, M.D.,
Bulletin of the Johns Hopkins Hospital, 1933

If it is practical, take someone with you to the doctor's office when discussing something this important. A friend or relative can help you with asking questions and with recording or remembering answers to those questions.

Think about and discuss all the information you have collected with a friend or family member. Ask yourself if the reasons given by your doctor for surgery seem logical. Give yourself time to reflect upon your reasoning and motivations in deciding for or against surgery. Ideally your decision should be based on a multitude of factors including your physical, social, emotional, and financial well-being.

You can also write or call the Vestibular Disorders Association and the Meniere's Network in the U.S. and similar organizations in other countries to get information about local support groups in your area and to find other people in your area who have similar problems. (See Chapter 39, "Where to Get More Information.") If you have a computer and modem, you can join groups discussing inner ear problems on the Internet. Keep in mind when doing this, that many people join these organizations because they have difficult problems; many people who could tell success stories have no need for a support group.

If you are thinking about surgery, examine your reasons carefully. Ask yourself the following questions:

• Do you look upon surgery as a quick fix for your problems?

• Do you feel that surgery is a sure thing or a permanent solution, always better than taking medicine or changing your diet?

• Do you think that things can't get any worse if you have surgery?

• Do you look upon surgery as a cure-all?

The four examples above are probably not good reasons to have surgery for Meniere's disease. First, some of the procedures are not a quick fix and require weeks to months for recuperation and to "get back to normal." As explained earlier, surgery for vertigo of any type is not a "sure thing." For some people, unfortunately, things can and do get worse with surgery. Finally, the surgery will probably not be a cure-all; none of the surgical procedures are thought to get rid of all symptoms and problems, particularly tinnitus and hearing loss.

If you have tried and failed to improve with a number of medical options, and the attacks of vertigo, hearing loss, tinnitus, and/or ear pressure are preventing you from being and feeling safe, engaging in social activities, taking care of yourself or others (children, spouse, parents), and/or working, and they are creating physical misery, surgery would seem to be a reasonable option to consider.

The Surgeries

The most commonly performed surgical procedures for Meniere's disease are the endolymphatic sac surgeries, labyrinthectomy, and vestibular nerve section.

Most otologists divide these inner ear surgeries for Meniere's disease into two categories, destructive and non-destructive. This categorization refers to the intent of the surgery, not to the outcome. The non-destructive surgery is aimed at changing the inner ear to make it work correctly again. The goal of destructive surgery is to stop the episodic vertigo by either destroying the inner ear itself or by cutting the balance nerve (both irreversible changes).

Note: Gentamicin treatments are discussed in Chapter 26, "Drugs Meant to Block Symptoms Permanently." Transtympanic dexamethasone treatments are discussed in Chapter 24, "Steroids."

Non-Destructive Surgery

Non-destructive surgery includes the many endolymphatic sac decompression procedures. These procedures are considered to be non-destructive because their goal is to improve the function of the inner ear by decreasing the amount of endolymph, not to destroy the inner ear or the nerve signal pathway to the brain. Even so, they involve cutting, leave scars, and can cause harm on occasion. Do not view the term "non-destructive" as meaning "can do no harm." Non-destructive simply means the intent of the surgery is not to destroy an area or a body function.

Endolymphatic sac decompression procedures (sometimes called endolymphatic sac enhancements) include:
• endolymphatic sac decompression
• endolymphatic sac-to-mastoid shunt
• endolymphatic sac-to-subarachnoid shunt
• endolymphatic valve
    Each of these procedures is done under general anesthesia and as

"same-day" surgery. They all include a C-shaped incision behind the ear, removal of much of the mastoid bone (mastoidectomy), and removal of temporal bone from around the endolymphatic sac.

In depth (anesthesia):
General anesthesia: You are given gas or intravenous drugs to cause and maintain a complete loss of consciousness. Usually you will have a tube down your throat so the anesthesiologist can "breathe for you" while you are unable to breathe on your own.
Regional anesthesia: An anesthetic is injected near a large collection of nerves or the spinal canal to "numb" a large area such as an arm or everything from the waist down.
Local anesthesia: An anesthetic agent is injected directly into the area in need of "deadening" such as a cut requiring stitches.
Topical anesthesia: An anesthetic agent is sprayed, poured, or rubbed onto an area in need of numbing such as the tympanic membrane.

The possible complications of these surgeries include hearing loss (can be total in almost five percent of all cases), increased tinnitus, increased amounts of vertigo, postoperative infection, cerebrospinal (spinal) fluid leak, and facial nerve damage.

These surgeries are supposed to decrease the amount of endolymph within the inner ear. Their intended outcome is to stop vertigo and to possibly improve hearing, reduce tinnitus, and reduce aural fullness. The episodes of vertigo have been reported to stop in as many as 50 to 60 percent of people having the surgery. (This is similar to the improvement rate reported for most treatments for Meniere's disease.)

Endolymphatic Sac Decompression

Endolymphatic sac decompression surgery is complete after the temporal bone has been removed from around the endolymphatic sac. Doctors using this procedure feel it increases circulation to the sac and increases endolymph absorption. It may also allow the sac to expand and reduce the endolymphatic pressure throughout the inner ear.

Endolymphatic Sac-to-Mastoid Shunt

After removing bone in the area, your surgeon inserts one end of a silastic tube or sheeting into the sac and the other end into the mastoid area. Doctors using endolymphatic sac-to-mastoid shunt surgery feel that excess endolymph will move from the inner ear to the mastoid cavity.

Endolymphatic Sac-to-Subarachnoid Shunt

During an endolymphatic sac-to-subarachnoid shunt surgery, the end of the silastic tubing draining endolymph away from the inner ear is placed into the subarachnoid space. This is a space filled with spinal fluid; the space lies between two of the three membranes protecting the brain. Doctors using this procedure feel that excess endolymph will drain from the inner ear into the subarachnoid space around the brain.

Endolymphatic Valve

Endolymphatic valve surgery involves insertion of a pressure release valve into the endolymphatic duct that leads from the inner ear to the endolymphatic sac. The other end of this device is in the mastoid cavity. Doctors using this believe that when endolymph pressure increases, the excess will be allowed to escape through the pressure release valve.

Controversy

Endolymphatic sac surgery is controversial; no well-controlled human studies have yet shown it to be effective. In fact, one European study comparing a group of people who had sac drainage to a group who had only a mastoidectomy claims to show that those who had sac drainage did less well than those who had only the mastoidectomy.

Some doctors feel that sac surgery works well and helps a significant number of people, while others feel it is no better than doing nothing. A selection of the wide ranging opinions from different otology journals appear below. (See the "References" section of this chapter for more complete information on the sources.)

> ". . . sac surgery in Meniere's disease should be regarded as an obsolete surgical procedure and discarded from the list of therapeutic measures in Meniere's disease."
> —C.R. Pfaltz, *Controversial Aspects of Meniere's Disease,* 1986

> "Endolymphatic sac surgery has a low morbidity and in the light of our current knowledge has a rational pathophysiological basis. It remains an extremely useful conservative surgical procedure and it would be a disservice to otology to cast it out of our armamentarium at this time."
> —D.A. Moffat, *Clinical Otolaryngology,* 1994

"The use of the endolymphatic subarachnoid shunt procedure performed early in the course of Meniere's disease can significantly reduce the risk of permanent hearing loss and disability."

—J.L. Pulec, *Acta Otolaryngologica, Supplement,* 1995

"If any hearing remains in the diseased ear, the first operation is an endolymphatic sac procedure."

—D.E. Brackmann, *Journal of Laryngology and Otology,*
1990

"The endolymphatic shunt operation did not significantly affect the long-term hearing results." (Written after comparing a group who did not have the surgery to a group who had it.)

—D.W. Goin, *et al.,*
American Journal of Otology, 1992

". . . these procedures provide only short-term preservation of hearing."

—J.R. Dickens and S.S. Graham,
American Journal of Otology, 1990

"Successful resolution of vertigo occurred in less than 60 percent [of people having one or another of the sac surgeries] at the Otology Group. Sac surgery therefore has been abandoned in favor of vestibular section for the surgical management of medically refractory Meniere's disease with disabling vertigo."

—M.E. Glasscock, *et al.,*
American Journal of Otology, 1989

Below is a personal account of an endolymphatic decompression procedure:

"I have suffered with Meniere's disease for 11 years now, although my symptoms were vastly improved by having a saccus decompression operation five years ago. However, I was plagued with periods of 'off' days consisting of muzzy heads, inability to concentrate, and fatigue."

—A.G., *Spin,* Autumn 1995

Destructive Surgery

The destructive surgeries for Meniere's disease include the labyrinthectomy and the vestibular nerve section.

Labyrinthectomy

A labyrinthectomy is the surgical removal of the balance end-organs within the saccule, utricle, and three ampullae of the semicircular canals, the parts of the inner ear that detect gravity and motion changes. There is general agreement that this procedure is highly effective in stopping violent episodes of vertigo caused by unilateral (one-sided) disease.

The intended outcome of the surgery is to prevent gravity and motion messages from reaching the brain from the side of the surgery and to stop the violent episodic vertigo of Meniere's disease. This procedure will cause deafness in the operated ear, and thus is only offered to someone with virtually no useful hearing left in the "bad" ear.

The severe episodes of vertigo stop in about 90 percent of the people having this surgery. The number having continued vestibular symptoms other than the specific episodes of vertigo is unclear. One study found that 50 percent of people undergoing the procedure did not return to work after the surgery.

The possible bad outcomes include facial nerve damage (temporary or permanent), infection that could involve the brain (thought to be rare), collection of blood under the skin (hematoma), increased tinnitus (could be permanent), no change in symptoms, taste disturbance and/or dry mouth (temporary or permanent), spinal fluid leak, and incomplete adjustment of the brain to the change in balance information.

The three types of labyrinthectomy are as follows:

• transcanal (done through the ear canal)

• transmastoid (done via an incision behind the ear followed by mastoidectomy—removal of the mastoid bone behind the ear)

• translabyrinthine vestibular nerve section (labyrinthectomy with removal of Scarpa's ganglion, a collection of nerve cell bodies found on the vestibular part of the vestibulo-cochlear nerve.)

General anesthesia is given for this procedure in all three forms. In the transcanal approach, the incision is made around the tympanic membrane within the ear canal and is only visible to an observer looking down the canal with an otoscope. In the transmastoid and translabyrinthine surgeries, hair is shaved from behind the ear, and an incision is made that will be visible after the surgery.

After this type of surgery, you will usually experience spinning vertigo, nausea, and/or vomiting until the brain begins to adjust (compensate) for the total loss of balance signals from one ear. (See Chapter 31, "Compensation.") The amount and severity of this vertigo will depend upon how much balance function was left in the operated ear. If an ear has little function, there will only be a small amount of vertigo after the surgery. It will usually be a few days before you will be able to walk without assistance or by hanging onto furniture and the walls.

Below is a description of the post-operative effects of this surgery, described by T.E. Cawthorne, *Journal of Laryngology and Otology*, 1943.

> "It is not necessary to describe in detail the nature of the post-operative disturbance; the typical picture of acute vestibular failure with the patient lying usually on his sound side, his head almost pushed into the pillow for support against the vertigo, a vomit bowl at hand, and the eyes closed. He dislikes any movement. . . . It is not uncommon when there is but little pre-operative function to find the patient lying on his back propped up with pillows and reading the paper the day after the operation."

Here is a personal account of labyrinthectomy:

> "After shunt surgery in July 1992, I had a wonderful remission that lasted for six months. Just as I was beginning to relax and trust that the nightmare was not coming back, it did come back 'out of the blue' one day. On March 13, 1996, I had a labyrinthectomy in my right ear. Thanks to God's mercy and my physician's skill, I have recovered very rapidly. No more dizziness or vertigo attacks. It is wonderful to be able to drive, take walks, shop, visit friends, make plans, and carry them out. I have rejoined the human race."
> —V.G., *On The Level*, Fall 1996

Vestibular Nerve Section

A vestibular nerve section cuts the vestibular branch of the vestibulo-cochlear nerve to prevent gravity and motion messages from reaching the brain and, thus, to stop the violent episodic vertigo of Meniere's disease on the side of the surgery.

Unlike a labyrinthectomy, this surgery does not destroy hearing. It is not, however, a treatment to improve or protect hearing, and hearing loss and deafness can occur as a complication in as many as 10 percent of the surgeries.

There are several types of nerve sections: retrolabyrinthine, middle fossa, retrosigmoid, suboccipital, and combination retrolabyrinthine/retrosigmoid.

General anesthesia is given for all forms of this procedure. Most of the surgeries include a C-shaped incision behind the ear. The incision for a middle fossa vestibular nerve section is made above the ear. Hair must be shaved from the operated area no matter which form of the procedure you have.

The vestibular nerve section surgery is different from both the endolymphatic procedures and the labyrinthectomies because it goes a bit beyond the inner ear and involves making an opening through the lining of the brain before cutting the vestibular branch of the vestibulo-cochlear nerve. Because of this, a neurosurgeon is usually involved, and you will spend time after the surgery in intensive care.

After this type of surgery, you will normally experience spinning vertigo and nausea/vomiting until your brain begins to adjust to (compensate for) the loss of balance signals from just one ear. (See Chapter 31, "Compensation.") The amount and severity of this vertigo will depend upon how much balance function was left in the operated ear. If an ear has little function, there will only be a small amount of vertigo after the surgery. Usually, a few days will pass before you will be able to walk without assistance.

The possible bad outcomes of a nerve section include hearing loss and/or deafness, facial nerve damage (temporary or permanent), spinal fluid leak, infection that could involve the brain (thought to be rare), collection of blood under the skin (hematoma), no change in symptoms, taste disturbance, dry mouth (temporary or permanent), and incomplete adjustment of the brain to the change in balance information.

The distinct episodes of vertigo stop in 90 to 95 percent of people having this surgery. It is unclear how many have continued vestibular symptoms other than episodic vertigo.

In depth (a problem area): Although most drawings of the vestibulo-cochlear nerve show completely separate cochlear and vestibular branches, in reality things are not so simple. Along a part of this nerve, including some areas where the surgery is done, the nerve has the appearance of one nerve rather than two branches, and fiber overlap sometimes occurs. A nerve section meant to sever only the vestibular fibers may miss some of them because they are not visibly separate from the cochlear fibers. (See Chapter 4, "Balance and the Other Vestibular Functions" and Figure 4-1, "Fiber Overlap," for more details.)

Vestibular Nerve Section—Personal Accounts

This first account is from a journal article about an Arizona physician whose attacks resumed about a year after having endolymphatic sac surgery. He decided to have a second surgery, a vestibular nerve section.

"Charlie's recovery from the second surgery, a selective sectioning of the right vestibular nerve, was much more difficult than the first. 'I had severe vertigo, was vomiting and couldn't stand or walk without assistance. I didn't quite comprehend the degree of difficulty the surgery would cause me,' he says. 'I don't remember much about my hospitalization. . . .'"

—*Barrow*, December 1992

The following account was originally published in *Spin*, the newsletter of the Meniere's Society of the United Kingdom. "MD" in the quote stands for Meniere's disease.

"I understand that my suitability for the proposed operation related to my age (49 at the time), my otherwise good level of fitness and health, the lack of any sign of MD in the other ear, and my lack of response to the various treatments already tried.

"It was explained to me that the proposed operation involved the cutting of the vestibular nerve. The neurosurgeon would locate the nerve and separate it from the hearing nerve, a delicate procedure considered to be important since I still had some hearing in that ear. The vestibular nerve contributed to balance, and the corresponding nerve in the other ear would take over the balance function for both sides. There would be a period of adjustment which might feel 'strange,' but the consultants found it difficult to describe, and I had not read about the operation or been able to talk with someone who had experienced it.

"My first response when waking from the operation was of dizziness and nausea, however this wore off. Over the next two days I gradually reached a sitting position, moving my head increasingly in a normal way. It was during this time that I noticed a feeling of slight unreality and light-headedness which can only be described as feeling mildly drunk! By the end of the second day, I was on my feet and there was a nurse available in case of loss of balance. In my first few steps, while I tried to head straight, I veered inadvertently to one side, but there was no real feeling of loss of balance. When I concentrated on going straight there was no problem. From then I experienced a re-learning process in all my movements. The light-headed feeling was present, and there was almost a tangible feeling of the remaining balance nerve taking over the function of the cut nerve. By the time I had left the hospital, five days after the operation, I had practiced all everyday movements—forward, backwards, turning, bending, stretching. Once or twice turning backwards quickly, I experienced momentary loss of balance, but it was of no real significance. "The re-routing process was quickly established, and reminders were there only when I did some unusual movement for the first time. The only movements I avoid are a jogging/jumping up and down type, which is visually uncomfortable.

"I can say that my experiences of this operation were in all ways positive. Four and a half years later, tinnitus remains and deafness progresses in that ear, but the devastating attacks are no longer there."

—*Spin*, Summer 1996 (with permission from the editor)

References

————. Barrow Neurological Institute. "Life with Meniere's Is a Balancing Act for Physician." *Barrow.* December 1992.

————. "Surgical Treatment of Incapacitating Peripheral Vertigo." *Otolaryngologic Clinics of North America,* 27(2):283-426. The entire April 1994 issue deals with surgery for Meniere's disease.

————. U.K. Meniere's Society. *Spin.* Autumn 1995 and Summer 1996.

Blakely, B.W., and Siegel, M.E. *Feeling Dizzy: Understanding and Treating Vertigo, Dizziness, and Other Balance Disorders.* New York: Macmillan, 1995.

Brackmann, D.E. "Surgical Treatment of Vertigo." *Journal of Laryngology and Otology,* 104:849-859, 1990.

Cawthorne, T.E. "The Treatment of Meniere's Disease." *Journal of Laryngology and Otology,* 58, 363-371, 1943.

Conn, H.F. *Current Therapy: Latest Approved Methods of Treatment for the Practicing Physician.* Philadelphia: W.B. Saunders Company, 1996.

Dandy, W.E. "Treatment of Meniere's Disease by Section of Only the Vestibular Portion of the Acoustic Nerve." *Bulletin of the Johns Hopkins Hospital,* 53:52-55, 1933.

Dandy, W.E. "The Surgical Treatment of Meniere's Disease." *Surgery, Gynecology, and Obstetrics,* 72:421-430, 1941.

Dickins, J.R., and Graham, S.S. "Meniere's Disease 1983-1989." *American Journal of Otology,* 11(1):51-65, 1990.

Fucci, M.J., Sataloff, R.T., and Myers, D.L. "Vestibular Nerve Section." *American Journal of Otolaryngology,* May-June: 15(3):180-9, 1994.

Glasscock, M.E., Jackson, C.G., Poe, D.S., and Johnson, G.C. "What I Think of Sac Surgery in 1989." *American Journal of Otology*, 10(3):230-233, 1989.

Goin, D.W., Mischke, R.E., Esses, B.A., Young, D., Priest, E.A., and Whitmayer-Goin, V. "Hearing Results from Endolymphatic Sac Surgery." *American Journal of Otology*, 13(5):393-397, 1992.

Green, J.D., Blum, D.J., and Harner, S.G. "Longitudinal Follow-Up of Patients with Meniere's Disease." *Otolaryngology-Head and Neck Surgery*, 104:783-788, 1991.

Huang, T.S., and Lin, C.C. "A Further Clinical Assessment of the Efficacy of Endolymphatic Sac Surgery." *Acta Otolaryngologica, Supplement*, 520:263-269, 1995.

LaRouere, M.J. "Surgical Treatment of Meniere's Disease." *Otolaryngologic Clinics of North America*, 29(2):311-321, 1996.

Moffat, D.A. "Endolymphatic Sac Surgery: Analysis of 100 Operations." *Clinical Otolaryngology*, 19:261-266, 1994.

Paparella, M.M. "Endolymphatic Enhancement." *Otolaryngologic Clinics of North America*, 27(2):381-401, 1994.

Pereira, K.D., and Kerr, A.G. "Disability After Labyrinthectomy." *Journal of Laryngology and Otology*, 110:216-218, 1996.

Pfaltz, C.R. *Controversial Aspects of Meniere's Disease.* New York: Thieme, Inc., 1986.

Pulec, J.L. "Surgical Treatment of Vertigo." *Acta Otolaryngologica, Supplement*, 519:21-25, 1995.

Rasmussen, A.T. "Studies of the VIIIth Cranial Nerve of Man." *Laryngoscope*, 50:67-83, 1940.

Rosenberg, S.I., Silverstein, H., Hoffer, M.E., and Thaler, E. "Hearing Results after Posterior Fossa Vestibular Neurectomy." *Otolaryngology Head and Neck Surgery,* 114:32-37, 1996.

Soderman, A.C., Ahlner, K., Bagger-Sjoback, D., and Bergenius, J. "Surgical Treatment of Vertigo — The Karolinska Hospital Policy (Stockholm, Sweden)." *American Journal of Otology*, 17:93-98, 1996.

Part V:
What You
Can Do

Life with Meniere's disease involves more than knowing symptoms, taking tests, and trying treatments.

Chapter 30

Prognosis

What Will Happen to Me?

The short answer to the question, "What will happen to me?" is that nobody knows.

Nobody can tell you with any degree of certainty what your future with Meniere's disease holds. Unfortunately no tests or rules can predict this accurately. The attacks of vertigo and other symptoms could stop tomorrow or go on for years. They could come sporadically or in clusters or groups; about 25 percent of the people with Meniere's disease experience attacks in clusters. They could also lessen, remain the same, or become more severe. Your second ear might become involved or might not; your hearing could improve, get worse, or fluctuate. The tinnitus could become more or less severe. A treatment might be found that will help you significantly, or you might improve without treatment.

> "The nature, intensity, direction, and duration of the attacks varied considerably, not only from patient to patient but also at times from attack to attack."
> —T.E. Cawthorne, *Annals of Otolaryngology—Head and Neck Surgery*, 1947

Although predictions specifically for you can't be made, you can learn a little about what the future could hold from others who have been in your situation. When large groups of people with Meniere's disease are studied over time, some patterns and tendencies emerge. This means that a large percentage, but never all, of the people with Meniere's disease will have some common experiences. The information presented below discusses these tendencies.

Can This Go Away?

No medication or treatment, even surgery, exists that has been proven to stop or fix the damage of endolymphatic hydrops, thought to be the inner ear change related to Meniere's disease. But some medications and treatments used in Meniere's disease are able to block or lessen the symptoms. The chance of requiring surgery or some other irreversible procedure to control vestibular symptoms is around 10 to 20 percent.

Will I Stay the Same?

The attacks of vertigo tend to go away with or without medical treatment.

> "Despite the cloud of pessimism which surrounds the treatment, we have found that in the majority of the patients who have come under our care it has been possible by one means or another to prevent or subdue attacks."
> —T.E. Cawthorne and A.B. Hewlett, *Proceedings of the Royal Society of Medicine*, 1954

> "Meniere's disease is in the great majority (86 percent) of cases a self-limiting disease. . . . The probable rate of cessation of attacks can be shown, namely that 70 percent will have ceased within one year."
> —B.H. Pickard, *Proceedings of the Royal Society of Medicine*, 1967

No way is known to accurately predict the length of attacks, their strength, or how often they will come, although it is thought the attacks are at their worst at the beginning of the disease. There are no "typical" number of attacks before the disease process stops or before there is nothing left undamaged within the inner ear (a situation sometimes referred to as "burnout"). In short, there is almost nothing typical about attacks of Meniere's disease, and this makes prediction impossible.

This disease is known for its variability not only from one person to the next but also from time to time within the same person. Nobody knows when the next attack will come, how strong it will be, when a long remission will present itself, how much hearing will be lost, or if the other ear will be affected. Even if the attacks occur frequently now, they could later decrease or stop. Long attacks could become shorter or stay the same.

The number, length, and strength of attacks in the future cannot be predicted. Your attacks could all stop tomorrow or continue for years. Violent attacks could simmer down; mild attacks could become stronger.

If the vertigo during an attack is extremely strong, there is no reason to think that a large hearing loss will also occur. On the other hand, the absence of severe attacks of vertigo does not guarantee minimal hearing loss.

What About My Hearing?

The presence of a fluctuating hearing loss is more common in the first few years of Meniere's disease, and a permanent level of loss is more common in later years. This loss usually stops at 50 to 60 decibels, less than total deafness; therefore, a hearing aid may be of benefit.

There is no way to predict how far a hearing loss will go. It is possible for Meniere's to cause deafness in the affected ear, and it is also possible that there might only be a minimal permanent hearing loss. Unfortunately there is no treatment option, including surgery, proven to stop or reverse hearing loss.

If the hearing loss becomes severe, hearing aids can help. If deafness or severe hearing loss were to occur in both ears, a cochlear implant (sometimes referred to as an artificial ear) might help with hearing as long as the cochlear nerve had not been cut or damaged by surgery or illness.

Tinnitus is also difficult to predict. Generally, however, as a hearing loss increases, the loudness of tinnitus also increases. However, most people are not as bothered later in Meniere's disease by tinnitus as they might have been in the earlier stages.

What About My Balance?

In the early stages of Meniere's disease, people generally do not experience balance difficulties such as staggering or balance symptoms such as feeling unsteady between attacks of vertigo (with the exception of the first couple of days after an attack). If the attacks occur far enough apart, the time between attacks should feel normal or nearly normal.

In the later stages of Meniere's disease or if both ears are involved, balance ability can become an issue. You may find it difficult to move comfortably in the dark and in visually confusing places.

What About the Other Ear?

A common worry for people with Meniere's disease is that the second ear will become involved. Indeed, it is possible to get Meniere's disease in the second ear. Statistics on this probability range from 12.6 percent to 77.8 percent, quite a spread. A study of people living in and around Rochester, Minn., between 1951 and 1980 found that 34.4 percent developed Meniere's in both ears. Studies looking at people for 10 years or longer seem to have the highest number of people with bilateral involvement as compared to studies of one to five years.

It is somewhat unusual to have Meniere's disease start in both ears at the same time or within six months of each other. If both ears are affected at the beginning, a strong possibility exists that the problem is something called autoimmune inner ear disease.

What If I Get Worse?

If your symptoms or situation worsen, tell your doctor. He or she will need your input to make correct treatment choices. In some cases where the quality of life has become a larger issue, more extreme treatment choices may be offered that were not offered earlier.

As the disease progresses to late-stage Meniere's disease, the attacks of vertigo usually decrease or disappear. The cessation of attacks is usually considered a relief that allows for an improvement in the quality of life.

Losing all or a great deal of the balance function in both ears does not force people into wheelchairs or to live out their lives in seclusion. The other two systems, the visual and proprioceptive, that are involved in balance can be relied on for walking and other aspects of balance. This is not as efficient as having the three systems working normally but can be many times better than having a malfunctioning vestibular system.

People with a large hearing loss from Meniere's disease can benefit from hearing aids, lip reading, and sign language just as any other person experiencing a hearing loss or deafness. Most big cities and many states have agencies with information and services for the hard of hearing or the deaf.

What About My Job?

The effect Meniere's disease will have on your ability to work is hard to determine, and few studies have been done that touch upon this topic. One study, done in Sweden, looked at 161 people with Meniere's disease, some for as long as 20 years, and found that the average number of work days lost each year because of Meniere's disease ranged from none to four.

If you can't work at your job, you may be covered by private disability insurance, and you can apply for Social Security disability payments. Whether you can get help through either of these depends on whether you meet the insurance or Social Security requirements. The personnel officer where you work, your insurance agent, and your local Social Security office staff should be able to help answer your questions about requirements.

Summary

Meniere's disease is incurable and not well understood. It is unpredictable, has no proven cure, can spread to the opposite ear, or can just stop on its own. Often the symptoms can be diminished or stopped with medical treatment. Most people with Meniere's disease improve over time and lead productive lives.

References

Cawthorne, T.E.. "Meniere's Disease." *Annals of Otolaryngology—Head and Neck Surgery*, 58:18-37, 1947.

Cawthorne, T.E., and Hewlett, A.B. "Meniere's Disease." *Proceedings of the Royal Society of Medicine*, 47:663-672, 1954.

Foxen, M. "The Use of Streptomycin in Meniere's Disease." *Proceedings of the Royal Society of Medicine*, 47:671-672, 1954.

Friberg, U., Stahle, J., and Svedberg, A. "The Natural Course of Meniere's Disease." *Acta Otolaryngologica*, 406:702-77, 1984.

Green, J.D., Blum, D.J., and Harner, S.G. "Longitudinal Follow-Up of Patients with Meniere's Disease." *Otolaryngology—Head and Neck Surgery*, 104:783-788, 1991.

Kitahara, M. "Bilateral Aspects of Meniere's Disease: Meniere's Disease with Bilateral Fluctuant Hearing Loss." *Acta Otolaryngologica, Supplement*, 485:74-77, 1991.

Kodama, K., Kitahara, M., and Kitanishi, T. "Clinical Findings in Meniere's Disease with Bilateral Fluctuant Hearing Loss." *Acta Otolaryngologica, Supplement.*, 519:227-229, 1995.

Paparella, M.M., and Griebie, M.S. "Bilaterality of Meniere's Disease." *Acta Otolaryngologica*, 97:233-237, 1984.

Pickard, B.H. "The Prognosis in Meniere's Disease." *Proceedings of the Royal Society of Medicine*, 60:968-969, 1967.

Shojaku, H., Watanabe, Y., Mizukoshi, K., Kitahara, M., Yazuwa, Y., Watanabe, I., and Ohkubo, J. "Epidemiological Study of Severe Cases of Meniere's Disease in Japan." *Acta Otolaryngologica*, 520:415-418, 1995.

Tokumasu, K., Fujino, A., Naganuma, H., Hoshina, I., and Araim, M. "Initial Symptoms and Retrospective Evaluation of Prognosis in Meniere's Disease." *Acta Otolaryngologica*, Supplement, 524:43-49, 1995.

Wladislavosky-Waserman, P., Facer, G.W., Mokrim, B., and Kurland, L.T. "Meniere's Disease: A 30-Year Epidemiological and Clinical Study in Rochester, Minn., 1951-1980." *Laryngoscope*, 94:1098-1102, 1984.

Chapter 31

Compensation

When a vestibular scientist or physician refers to compensation, he or she is talking about the brain's adjustment to loss of motion-and-gravity signals from the inner ear. The purpose of compensation is to eliminate spatial disorientation and dizziness and re-establish optimal balance function and the clearest vision possible. In most cases, dizziness will be absent and balance and vision will seem nearly normal to you after compensation has occurred.

Compensation is usually of concern to someone with Meniere's disease when he or she is undergoing a treatment such as transtympanic gentamicin, vestibular nerve section, or labyrinthectomy that will produce loss of function on one side of the vestibular system. If compensation did not exist, the "destructive" treatments for Meniere's disease would both relieve the episodes of strong vertigo and leave a permanent balance disability that would reduce the quality of life significantly. Instead, because of compensation, removing all function on the "bad" side can improve things significantly in someone having frequent, incapacitating attacks of vertigo.

Compensation can also occur after an attack of Meniere's disease especially when several weeks go by between attacks. Attacks occurring more often than once a month often do not allow the body enough time to compensate. Compensation can also be more difficult as you get older.

The word "compensation" sounds like a simple and straightforward process whereby one side of the vestibular nuclei in the brain takes over for the side with reduced or absent function. However, scientists carrying out studies of the vestibular system have determined that one side does not just take over for both sides. Other areas of the brain, body sensors, and eye-movement systems, substitution with vision and proprioception, and factors that may not yet have been discovered join to compensate for the lost vestibular function.

Of course, the important thing for someone who has lost vestibular function is that life can get back to normal, and knowing which systems and areas of the body are responsible may not be of much interest. However, if compensation does not occur and a person's function does not return to normal, it can be helpful to understand the areas and systems responsible for compensation.

Stages

Compensation begins immediately after a loss of vestibular function whether it occurs because of disease or as the result of treatment. Compensation reduces the nystagmus and vertigo experienced after a labyrinthectomy and vestibular nerve section and allows walking within a day or two of the loss and resumption of normal activities within six weeks to several months.

There are two stages in compensation, acute, also called static or tonic compensation, and chronic, also called dynamic compensation.

Acute compensation occurs spontaneously in the first few days after a change or loss and is responsible for slowing or stopping the nystagmus, vertigo, vomiting, body sway, and the need to stand with the feet further apart than usual. Within a week, there should be no spontaneous nystagmus when the eyes are open in a lighted room, and the other symptoms present when the head is still should be nearly gone.

Unlike acute compensation, chronic compensation after a loss is not automatic. It is engaged by active movement involving the head and the use of vision. It usually becomes the most complete when lots of intentional movement has occurred and intentional vision has been used. Satisfactory chronic compensation helps to reinstate efficient muscle use, stops instability during head turns, and stops the odd symptoms caused by movements such as walking. Chronic compensation can take six weeks for some people and up to several months in others, and the degree of its success depends on various factors.

Factors That Help Chronic Compensation

Younger people in good physical condition who have undergone a slow reduction in vestibular function have the easiest and most complete compensation. Older people, particularly those over age 65, usually have the most difficulty after losing vestibular function.

Many activities such as moving the head, walking, watching moving objects, looking at objects while moving the head, moving the head while looking at moving objects, and walking in places that are visually "busy" can all aid in fully establishing compensation.

Chronic compensation can, in some situations, be sped up and made more complete by an organized program of exercises developed by a physical therapist.

Drugs have also been shown in some animal studies to speed up compensation, but drugs are generally not used in humans to aid compensation. Actually many drugs hinder compensation as noted below.

Factors Hindering Compensation

Several factors can prevent or slow down compensation including insufficient use of vision (for example, keeping the eyes closed or not watching any moving scenes), immobility (for example, staying in bed too much or rigidly holding the head to avoid movement), use of sedatives such as Dramamine and Valium, a history of alcohol abuse, diabetes mellitus, neck and back pain, hypertension, brain concussion, and history of exposure to industrial solvents at work. Advanced age and poor physical conditioning can also interfere with compensation.

Failure to Compensate

Not everyone losing vestibular function on one side will compensate or compensate fully. Some reasons for this failure include the following:

- The treatment did not stop all signals from leaving the problem ear and arriving in the brain.
- Age-related changes have occurred in the nervous system.
- The "healthy" side also has a problem.
- Medications may have prevented compensation.
- You have a problem in the cerebellum or some other critical area of the brain.
- Significant problems with back or neck or limb sensation or pain have occurred.
- Something occurred during the critical time in which compensation usually takes place that stopped or prevented the process.
- You have not moved enough or are unable to move enough for compensation to occur.

Loss of Compensation

Chronic compensation is also called dynamic compensation because it is a constantly changing entity. Once compensation is achieved, it may not be permanent. A loss of compensation, also called decompensation, can occur. Fatigue, illness, stress, fluctuating function in the remaining ear, a period of inactivity, a change in medication, anesthesia, and some drugs can cause temporary decompensation. The drugs that can cause decompensation include alcohol, tranquilizers, strong pain medications, muscle relaxants, and anti-nausea, anti-vertigo, anti-vomiting and anticonvulsant preparations (the same drugs that can hinder compensation).

When the situation resolves, activity is resumed, or the drugs are stopped, compensation should re-establish itself.

Summary

Your brain can adjust for one-sided function loss through compensation and provide you with better balance function and clearer vision.

References

Baloh, R.W., and Halmagyi, G.M. *Disorders of the Vestibular System.* New York: Oxford University Press, 1996.

Black, F.O., Wade, S.W., and Nashner, L.M. "What Is the Minimal Vestibular Function Required for Compensation?" *American Journal of Otology,* 17:401-409, 1996.

Curthoys, I.S., and Halmagyi, G.M. "Vestibular Compensation: A Review of the Oculomotor, Neural, and Clinical Consequences of Unilateral Loss." *Journal of Vestibular Research,* 5(2) 67-107, 1995.

Jackler, R.K., and Brackmann, D.E. *Neurotology.* St. Louis: C.V. Mosby Company, 1994.

Shepard, N.T., and Telian, S.A. *Practical Management of the Balance Disorder Patient.* San Diego, California: Singular Publishing Group, Inc., 1996.

Yamanaka, T., Sasa, M., Amano, T., Miyahara, H., and Matsunaga, "The Role of Glucocorticoid in Vestibular Compensation in Relation to Activation of Vestibular Nucleus Neurons." *Acta Otolaryngologica, Supplement,* 519:168-172, 1995.

Chapter 32

Coping

People have found many ways to cope with Meniere's disease. Like everyone else, you must discover what works for you.

Many sources offer advice on how to avoid or stop attacks and to reduce stress. However, Meniere's varies so much from case to case that little advice is universally useful. For example, one pamphlet on Meniere's disease suggests that avoiding sudden movements may help prevent dizziness. This is appropriate during the attack phase of the Meniere's cycle but inappropriate during the remission phase, when movement may help the vestibular system and brain to adjust. Discuss coping advice with your physician to get a better idea of its fitness for your particular case.

This chapter includes a variety of coping tips. Other tips appear in Chapter 33, "Safety," and Chapter 34, "Preservation, Protection."

General Tips

To help cope with your Meniere's disease, keep yourself fit through good diet, exercise, and adequate sleep. Good balance requires strong muscles, flexible joints, and an alert mind.

Learn all you can about Meniere's disease, as suggested by E. F. in the following comment in *Spin* (Spring 1996), the newsletter of the United Kingdom Meniere's Society.

> "Can you learn to control the disease and not let it control you? Well, I think you can to some extent. First, I feel it's important to learn all you can about MD. Read books, talk to fellow sufferers. Question the doctors and consultants, and of course learn from the Meniere's Society. Do not accept tablets or treatments without understanding how they work. You know your body better than anyone else, and it's you who has to suffer any side effects. So question the professionals; then you feel more in control of what is happening to you."

Try some of these coping strategies suggested by the New South Wales (Australia) Meniere's Support Group (as reprinted in *Spin*):

- Rest when you feel tired.
- Listen to a relaxation or meditation tape upon waking each morning and just before retiring at night.
- Go for a 20-minute brisk walk each day. If you don't feel confident about going alone, ask someone to go with you. Use a walking stick if necessary.
- Reduce caffeine intake.
- Avoid salt and too much sugar. Read labels carefully for sodium (salt) and sugar content.
- Keep a diary of your activities and what you have eaten. Allergies, especially to foods, may cause an increase in body fluids and increase your vestibular symptoms.
- Wear flat shoes as much as possible.
- Place night lights where you are likely to go during the night.
- Avoid noisy, crowded situations.
- Instead of going out, invite friends to your place, where you can control your surroundings.
- Avoid smoking.
- Avoid alcohol.
- Ask your family to learn about Meniere's disease to help them understand why your behavior changes during and after an attack.
- Face people when they talk to you. Ask them not to shout, since loud noise is stressful, and shouts become distorted.
- Join a support group, and keep up with the latest medical findings.
    When traveling by car during cold weather, be prepared for a winter emergency. Keep drinking water, a blanket or sleeping bag, and pocket- or hand-warmers in your car. (The latter can be found in stores with camping or hunting departments.)

Preparing for Vomiting, Diarrhea

- Request a prescription for an anti-vomiting drug in the form of a rectal suppository, which eliminates the possibility of vomiting the medicine.
- Ask your doctor ahead of time at what point you should seek help; for example, after 12 hours of vomiting and of not eating or drinking.
- Keep an electrolyte replenisher like Gatorade on hand to prevent dehydration and mineral imbalance. Ask your doctor about when to use such fluids.
- Carry plastic bags (for vomiting), mouth wash, breath mints, and a change of clothes with you when you travel.

- Have a basin or empty garbage can available in your bathroom (if your usual habit is to get to the bathroom).
- Have room deodorizer available.
- If you know you will not be able to get to a bathroom, keep an adult diaper or a towel and large garbage can liner on hand.

Warning Phase Tips

- If you experience warning symptoms, locate any medicine you may require and take as directed by your doctor.
- If you are driving, pull off the road.
- If you are alone, check the kitchen to make sure the stove top and oven are turned off.
- Empty your bladder and, if convenient, your bowel.
- On a hot day, don't leave an air-conditioned building to seek refuge and privacy in your car parked outside. You might overheat in the car and endanger yourself.
- Change into something more comfortable (if possible).

Attack Phase Tip

Little can be done to stop a spontaneous attack of violent vertigo from occurring. Take drugs as prescribed. Staying put, moving slowly, or moving the body carefully are the best courses of action until the vertigo stops.

General Communication Tips

- Have a phone with a speed-dialing capability to get help at the touch of a button.
- If you often travel alone by car or are otherwise away from buildings and other people, a cell phone might be a good investment.
- A great many people with Meniere's disease find that discussing their symptoms and problems with others is beneficial. This can be done in person, via telephone, through regular mail, and via the Internet.

"During the beginning of my spells, I did not know of any support groups. The loneliness of the illness gripped me. When the second series of attacks arrived, I was aware of the groups. It was a much easier siege to handle. The fact that there are people out there to help and go along with your spells was the only bonus one could have. It seems so much easier to cope when others are having the same feelings. The friends I have met through the networks are worth more than I could ever express."

—B.L., letter to the author, 1996

• Use the Internet or on-line services to meet people if you are having trouble communicating and/or socializing with people in person or by telephone.

"The real beauty of the Internet however, for someone who is hard of hearing, is that you can be in instant contact with a potential 30 million people worldwide sharing ideas, asking questions, and just communicating with like-minded souls, without having to struggle with a telephone, apologize for asking them to repeat themselves all the time, or pretend you're following what they are saying, when you aren't."

—*Spin*, Summer 1996

For more information on how to find other people with Meniere's disease, see Chapter 39, "Where to Get More Information."

Other Tips

Reading

• Use a non-flickering light source. Don't try to read with a fluorescent light or from the light generated by your TV or computer monitor.
• Move from word to word by placing your finger under each word to help keep your eyes on the right spot.
• Place a ruler (a solid ruler, not one you can see through) under the sentence you are trying to read.
• Read in a place that is quiet and visually calm.

Bothersome Bright Lights

• While you are outdoors, wear sunglasses that block glare. Use a sun hat, sun visor, or baseball cap to supplement the sunglasses.

"I purchased wrap-around sunglasses closed in at the top, too. It made life a lot easier. I could not be in the light without them."

—R.C., letter to the author, 1997

Poor Depth Perception

• On an overcast day, try wearing glasses that are yellow or amber.

One-Sided Deafness; Severe Hearing Loss

- Tell people who must interact with you about your hearing loss so they will not think you are ignoring them.
- All sounds will seem to come from your normal or more normal side, so get into the habit of looking around to determine the direction a sound is coming from. Don't assume that you can figure this out with just one ear.

Increased Sound Sensitivity

- Avoid bothersome sound when you can.
- A combination of ear muffs and ear plugs can keep out some unwanted sounds. When you use these, be vigilant for people trying to talk to you.

Tinnitus

Tinnitus can be covered up or masked by a fan, radio static, or anything with a constant sound. "White-noise" machines, also called sleep-sound generators, may help you sleep. You might also use a tinnitus masker during the day. Ask your audiologist about these devices.

> "Over the years I have found that the best way of controlling, or should I say ignoring, my tinnitus is to become thoroughly absorbed in an interesting pastime. For me this has to be the construction of scale model ships."
> —B.L., *Spin*, June 1995

Difficulty Writing

- Write important things when you are well rested and without distractions.
- If what you are writing is really important, find someone to proofread it for you.

Poor Memory

- Make notes about things you want to remember, or use a tape recorder.
- Use "cheat" sheets when appropriate.

Muscle and Joint Tightness or Pain

- Get adequate exercise (Always check with your personal physician before undertaking an exercise program.)

- Stress reduction and relaxation methods might be of benefit, particularly if stress itself is causing the tightness or pain.

Difficulty Walking Straight; Staggering

- Use cues from your surroundings about the location of horizontal and vertical.
- Walk along a wall rather than in the open.
- Wear flat shoes with non-skid soles.
- Pick something in the distance to walk towards.

Fatigue

- Go at a slower pace around the time of an attack, and if attacks occur often, use a slow pace as much as needed.
- Get help when you need it.
- Because stress can lead to fatigue, reduce it as much as possible. (See "Stress Control" later in this chapter.)
- Allow yourself enough time to get adequate sleep at night; you may need to make this a priority.
- Eat a well-balanced and adequate diet.
- Exercise regularly.
- Depression can lead to fatigue. If you think you might be depressed, get help from your primary care physician or a mental health professional.

Loss of Self-Confidence and Self-Esteem

- Take control as best you can.
- Prepare for any situation you can predict.
- Learn all about your disease and the treatment you are undergoing.
- Be involved in your care.
- Set your own goals. Don't automatically use those of your peers or of society.
- Determine your priorities.
- When you are able, look for the positives in your life and in your experience with Meniere's disease.

> "I am a much better doctor because of the Meniere's and subsequently because of being a patient."
>
> —C.D., *Barrow,* 1992

Fear

When you feel afraid, try to determine exactly what you fear. If you can identify the fear precisely, you may be able to lessen it. For example, if you have a big fear of vomiting, discuss with your doctor the possibility of having a prescription anti-vomiting drug on hand at all times, just in case.

Stress Control

Many articles, videotapes, audiotapes, and books discuss stress, how to use it, or how to lessen it. The approach to stress outlined below is just one of many.

Here are three steps to mastering the stress in your life:

1) Recognize your symptoms of stress. Tune in to your body, listen to what it is telling you. Do you have warning signals? Does your head ache? Do you feel tension in the back of your neck? By heeding these signals, you can recognize that stress is beginning to affect you.

2) Identify the sources of your stress. Sometimes you can handle big problems more easily than everyday ones. Worrying about little things wastes lots of energy.

3) Take action. What can you do to change? Promote your health by eating better, by getting adequate rest and exercise, and by following medical advice. Cut down on the unnecessary, and do the most important things first. Being actively involved with a support group may be helpful. Don't be afraid to reach out for help.

Your personal philosophy of life can make a difference. Openly communicate with friends. Learn to laugh. A sense of humor is an excellent coping mechanism. Take responsibility for the stress in your life.

Summary

Advice and tips are available from many sources for making life with Meniere's disease easier. By picking and choosing appropriately, you may be able to improve your life.

References

_____. Barrow Neurological Institute. "Life with Meniere's Is a Balancing Act for Physician." *Barrow*, December 1992.

_____. U.K. Meniere's Society, *Spin*, June 1995, Spring 1996, Summer 1996.

238 ❖ *Meniere's Disease—What You Need to Know*

Farber, S.D. "Living with Meniere's Disease: An Occupational Therapist's Perspective." *American Journal of Occupational Therapy*, 43(5): 341-343, 1989.

Chapter 33

Safety

S afety can be a big concern for many people with Meniere's disease. A hearing loss can be a problem, and so can vestibular symptoms, particularly vertigo. Safety issues may concern not only someone with Meniere's but other people as well; for example, those who might be injured in a car crash with someone having a Meniere's attack. Safety issues may also concern law officers, insurance companies, and government agencies.

While it's true that Meniere's disease doesn't normally cause damage except to the inner ear, having an attack at a bad time or place could put you and other people at risk for serious harm. Constantly thinking about the next attack of Meniere's disease is not a good idea; however, it's wise to identify safety concerns and to be prepared.

Preparing means asking your doctor about the safety of driving and performing activities you might usually engage in such as climbing ladders, hiking in the back of beyond, or bicycling. If you have to decide on your own what activities are safe or how to make your activities safer, you should consider:

- the amount of time you normally have between warning symptoms and attack
- symptoms such as vertigo, fatigue, blurry vision, nausea, bouncing vision, jerking/jumping vision, or visually stimulated disorientation that occur before, during, and after attacks
- activities that interest you, including requirements and location

Your doctor will not be able to make every decision for you about safety concerns. Only you know how well or poorly you are feeling, what your capabilities have been, and what level of confidence you have in your present abilities. For example, if you feel too sick to drive, don't do it.

Hearing Loss

A hearing loss can go far beyond a simple annoyance. It can cause a driver at an intersection to overlook an oncoming fire truck, make it impossible to know the direction of a honking horn, or make emergency instructions hard to hear.

Deafness or a large hearing loss in one ear can make it impossible to determine the direction a noise is coming from. Hearing loss or hearing loss combined with noise from a car radio or stereo can limit your ability to hear audio clues to problems on the road.

If you have a hearing loss, don't play the car radio or stereo too loudly. Pay close visual attention to the road for emergency vehicles, cars, and people you may not hear.

Listen closely when being given instructions such as those that flight attendants give on airplanes. Ask for a repeat if you don't understand what has been said. Get and wear a medic alert tag that lists your hearing loss. (You can write to a non-profit organization called MedicAlert at 2323 Colorado Ave., Turlock, CA 95382, for details, or call them at 1-800-763-3428.)

Hearing loss has been implicated in one study as a possible factor in traffic accidents. The authors found that people over age 65 who were involved in car crashes were twice as likely as normal to have been using a hearing aid at the time of the accident.

Drop Attacks

If you begin having drop attacks (Tumarkin's otolithic crises), report them to your doctor as soon as possible. A drop attack is one of the few ways that Meniere's disease can and does cause serious bodily harm. Because you have no warning before a drop attack, you will fall into whatever is beneath you. You could break your neck or sustain a serious head injury. (See Chapter 12, "Late-Stage Meniere's Disease," for more on drop attacks, which can occur at any stage of Meniere's disease but are somewhat more common late in the disease process.)

Drug Effects

The drugs used to treat Meniere's disease and its symptoms can cause a number of side effects, many of which could affect safety. Blurred vision, sleepiness, slowed reaction times, and slow decision-making can create danger in many activities such as taking a shower, slicing food in the kitchen, cutting wood with a chain saw, operating power tools, driving a car, and anything else that requires alertness and hand-eye coordination.

Many times these symptoms abate over time as the body adjusts to the presence of the drug(s). When first starting any course of drug treatment, be particularly careful in all your activities until you learn how the drug affects you.

Some evidence indicates that people over 65 years old who are taking anti-anxiety drugs have a 45 percent higher rate of traffic accidents during the first week they take the drugs and a 25 percent higher rate overall than do people over 65 years who are not taking the drugs. Other evidence suggests that seniors on antidepressants have an increased chance of being in an automobile accident. And other research suggests that people age 55 and older taking a benzodiazepine (Valium, Xanax, Ativan) have a larger chance of falling and breaking a thigh bone than people not taking one of these drugs.

Driving

When thinking about your fitness to drive, put safety ahead of need or desire. Many symptoms from both the ear and from drugs can impair the ability to drive. These include blurred vision, bouncing vision, sleepiness/fatigue, slowed reaction time, positioning vertigo (head movement vertigo), visually stimulated disorientation and/or vertigo, mental distraction, and distortion of lights, such as headlights, in darkness.

> "Because the onset of my Meniere's is usually so rapid and violent at best, I only drive around our neighborhood (never on a highway). My rule of thumb is that I will drive around the neighborhood after my vision has been clear for a week."
> —B.K., letter to author, 1996

No studies have been published about being distracted by vestibular sensations while driving, but one study revealed a connection between another kind of distraction and car wrecks. The study found that people who use cell phones while driving have a quadrupled chance of having an accident. (This statistic held true even for drivers using cell phones not held to the ear by hand.)

The law may also have something to say about Meniere's and your driving. Government rules dealing with fitness to drive differ from state to state, province to province, and country to country. For example, the Canadian Medical Association publishes a "Physician Guide to Driver Examination" that includes a few passages relevant to Meniere's disease:

> "Patients with recurrent peripheral disorders (i.e., Meniere's disease), who are subject to unexpected attacks of vertigo, should not drive any class of motor vehicle until their symptoms have been controlled.

> "Patients with permanent unilateral loss of vestibular function may drive any type of motor vehicle after compensation has been established, which usually takes a few weeks. However, those with bilateral loss of function or loss of func-

tion due to brainstem disease should not be allowed to drive at all."

Piloting an Aircraft

For piloting an aircraft, fewer grey areas exist than for driving, and only one agency regulates the skies above the entire U.S., the Federal Aviation Agency (FAA). Its regulations concerning first-, second-, and third-class aviators include requirements for medical certification. One of these denies certification to an aviator with a "disease or condition manifested by, or that may reasonably be expected to be manifested by, vertigo or a disturbance of equilibrium."

It follows from this requirement that someone with Meniere's disease should not be piloting an aircraft and cannot be medically cleared to fly in the U.S. even if currently licensed.

Safety During the Meniere's Cycle

Warning

People with a pre-attack warning know when an attack is about to occur. This warning can allow time to stop an activity and find a safe place to stay during the attack. Driving, for instance, can most likely be done safely since you can pull off the road before an attack. On the other hand, a vacation in the Himalayas or deep in Yellowstone National Park may not be safe since you may not have enough time after the warning to take shelter from dangerous weather.

If you have no warning and your attacks come entirely out of the blue, many activities such as driving, swimming, sky diving, scuba diving, piloting an airplane, or climbing a ladder could result in severe injury or death. In some cases, the danger extends to other people who might be hurt if, for example, you lost control of a car or plane.

Attack

Attacks of Meniere's disease can vary widely from person to person and sometimes from one attack to the next in the same person. If the attacks are short and mild and merely cause you to sit down for a while, you might not need to stop wilderness hiking trips, or water skiing, or other adventurous or vigorous pursuits.

However, even people who experience only mild attacks should not do any activities requiring hand-eye coordination or balance during the attack. You should not drive during even a mild attack because of disturbed vision, slowed reaction time, and the general feeling of "being sick."

When attacks last hours and cause considerable vertigo, nausea, vomiting, sweating, and the like, many activities may become potentially hazardous. The availability of a dry, warm, protected place to ride out an attack must be considered. A cross-country skiing trip deep into the Colorado Rockies, for example, could become deadly if an attack were to occur on a trail miles from shelter during a snow storm. Activities such as bowling or playing softball would not involve the same risk.

Aftermath

During the aftermath of an attack, many people are extremely tired, sleepy, have problems with visually stimulated disorientation and vertigo, have positioning vertigo, or other "odd" sensations when they move their head, and they may feel a little bit tipsy. During this period, reaction time may be slowed; hand-eye coordination may be off a bit, and walking or standing may be difficult.

The aftermath is not the time to drive a car, climb a ladder, operate equipment or machinery, cross a busy road on foot, or take a shower. Walking any place with an uneven or slippery surface might cause a fall.

Walking around, moving your head, washing dishes, vacuuming the house, typing, gardening, washing the car, and other low-risk activities usually help get things back to normal in the period after an attack.

Coping Strategies

Try to prepare for things that could go wrong if you were disabled by an attack and its aftermath during your activities. If you have stopped going on long walks or bicycle rides because you fear having an attack and getting stranded, a cell phone might be the solution. Exercising with a partner would also work. Carrying a whistle that could be used to get attention if you are stranded might also work.

Long out-of-town car rides can also cause a good deal of worry. Again, a cell phone could be used to summon help if needed. If you are concerned about being stranded in a cold car in winter, keep warm clothes, blankets, or a sleeping bag in the car as well as a cell phone.

Summary

Safety is a concern for many people with Meniere's disease. Many activities are safe; others are safe under certain conditions, while others may never be safe.

Other tips related to safety can be found in Chapter 34, "Preservation, Protection."

References

Baloh, R.W., and Halmagyi, G.M. *Disorders of the Vestibular System.* New York: Oxford University Press, 1996.

Federal Aviation Administration. "Federal Aviation Regulations." http://www.safetydata.com/far-67.htm. Oct. 30, 1997.

Hemmelgarn, B., Suissa, S., Huang, A., Boivin, J.F., and Pinard, G. "Benzodiazepine Use and the Risk of Motor Vehicle Crash in the Elderly." *Journal of the American Medical Association,* 278:27-31, 1997.

Herings, R.M., Stricker, B.H., DeBoer, A., Bakker, A., and Sturmans, F. "Benzodiazepines and the Risk of Falling Leading to Femur Factures: Dosage More Important Than Elimination Half-Life." *Archives of Internal Medicine,* 155(16):1801-1807, 1995.

Leveille, S.G., Buchner, D.M., Koepsell, T.D., McCloskey, L.W., Wold, M.E., and Wagner, E.H. "Psychoactive Medications and Injurious Motor Vehicle Collisions Involving Older Drivers." *Epidemiology,* 5(6):591-598, 1994.

McCloskey, L.W., Koepsell, T.D., Wolf, M.E., and Buchner, D.M. "Motor Vehicle Collision Injuries and Sensory Impairments of Older Drivers. *Ageing,* 23(4):267-273, 1994.

Parnes, L.S., and Sindwani, R. "Impact of Vestibular Disorders on Fitness to Drive: A Census of the American Neurotology Society." *American Journal of Otology,* 18:79-85, 1997.

Redelmeier, D.A., and Tibshirani, R.J. "Association Between Cellular Telephone Calls and Motor Vehicle Collisions." *New England Journal of Medicine,* 336(7):453-458, 1997.

Chapter 34

Preservation, Protection

S ince the cause of Meniere's disease is unknown, no one knows how to prevent it. However, you can protect your hearing and balance from factors unrelated to Meniere's disease.

You can develop habits to prevent damage to the ears, vestibulo-cochlear nerve, brain, eyes, proprioceptors (pressure sensors located in the joints), muscles, and joints. You can also be aware of situations and substances that can cause temporary balance difficulties by their impact on vestibular function, vision, proprioception, alertness, and the muscles and joints, and you can make wise decisions based on that knowledge.

Infection, noise trauma, pressure changes, poisoning (drugs and chemicals), general trauma, and drugs can all affect hearing and balance.

Ears Only

Noise Trauma

Loud noise can cause damage to the cochlea and produce hearing loss and/or tinnitus. Some research also suggests that noise can affect the vestibular (balance) parts of the ear.

Hearing damage can begin to occur when you are exposed to nois-es over 70 decibels. Table 34-1 shows noise exposure guidelines pub-lished by the Occupational Safety and Health Administration (OSHA) of the U.S. Federal government.

Table 34-1: OSHA Noise Exposure Guidelines for Workers			
Decibels (dB)	Hours	Decibels (dB)	Hours
0	8	102	1½
92	6	105	1
95	4	110	½
97	3	115	¼
100	2		

Steps you can take to protect your ears:

- Stay away from loud noise.
- Be aware of decibel levels. Anything over 70 can cause damage, and it is cumulative; that is, it adds up over time.
- Avoid constant exposure to leaf blowers, vacuums, hair driers, heavy motorized machinery, guns, pistols, rifles, loud stereo head phones, drills, chain saws, snowmobiles, jack hammers, sandblasting, jet aircraft, rock concerts and similar things that produce loud noise.
- Use ear plugs/ear muffs when loud noise can't be avoided (plugs to block low-pitched sounds and muffs to block high-pitched sounds).

Caution: The use of ear plugs and ear muffs make hearing and understanding speech difficult for people with a hearing loss.

Pressure Changes

Activities that create large pressure changes such as blowing your nose with both nostrils closed, trying to squelch a sneeze, scuba diving, sky diving, or flying in an unpressurized airplane or helicopter have all been implicated in causing damage to structures in the middle ear that can affect hearing and/or balance.

Steps you can take:

- Beware of changing ear pressure drastically and quickly.
- Blow your nose gently, with one nostril open.
- Don't try to stop a sneeze in progress.
- Don't ride in an unpressurized aircraft.
- Consult your physician before sky diving or scuba diving.
- If you find that flying brings on symptoms such as vertigo, hearing loss, increased tinnitus or fullness, discuss it with your doctor and try to travel some other way. Don't try to "get used to it."

Ototoxins

An ototoxin is an ear poison. Oto=ear, and toxin=poison. Many drugs and chemicals, from aspirin to xylene, can be ototoxic. Damage from these substances may involve hearing (cochleotoxicity) or balance (vestibulotoxicity) and can be temporary or permanent. It has been suggested that the presence of Meniere's disease may increase the risk of damage from an ototoxin.

Cochleotoxicity can cause tinnitus, aural pressure, and/or hearing loss. Vestibulotoxicity can cause general unsteadiness, visual difficulty, possible oscillopsia, and other symptoms. Vertigo is not usually experienced.

Members of five drug groups cause the majority of diagnosed oto-toxicity cases. These are the salicylates (the drug family aspirin belongs to), quinines, loop diuretics, aminoglycoside antibiotics, and some anti-neoplastics (anti-cancer drugs). Some other antibiotics and a large group of chemicals that don't fit into a single group can also be ototoxic.

Acetylsalicylic acid, often abbreviated ASA, is the formal name for aspirin. All the salicylates, including aspirin and others such as magnesium salicylate and sodium salicylate, are potential ototoxins. (See Table 34-2 for the names of many drugs containing salicylates.) As many as 11 out of every 1,000 people taking aspirin develop cochleotoxicity, almost always temporary.

Table 34-2: Some Drugs Containing Salicylates

Alka-Seltzer	Astrin	Entrophen	Salgesic
Amigesic	Cosprin	Hiprin	Salsitab
Anacin	Diagen	Magan	Supasa
Ancasal	Disalcid	Measurin	Triaphen-10
Arthra-G	Doan's	Mobidin	Tricosal
Arthritis Pain	Easprin	Mono-Gesia	Trilisate
Formula	Ecotrin	Mono-Gesic	Uracel
Arthropan	Empirin	Novase	ZORprin
Aspergum	Encaprin	Salflex	

The quinines are fairly common. They can be found in prescription form, over-the-counter, and in the tonic water readily available at the neighborhood grocery store. Quinines are also used, unfortunately, to "cut" heroin. They can be found in some heart drugs, anti-malaria drugs, and leg cramp drugs. (See Table 34-3, next page, for names of some quinine drugs.) Quinine ototoxicity causes temporary damage to the cochlea and has also been associated with temporary vestibular malfunction.

Loop diuretics are known to cause temporary cochleotoxic problems on occasion. These drugs are ethacrynic acid (Edecrin), furosemide (Lasix), bumetanide (Bumex), and torsemide (Demedex).

Aminoglycoside antibiotics are a group of strong drugs given mostly by injection or intravenously. Some members of the group are cochleotoxic, some are vestibulotoxic, and others can be both. (See Table 34-4, next page.)

A handful of anti-cancer drugs can cause permanent cochlear damage. (See Table 34-5, page 251.)

Erythromycin, given intravenously, can cause temporary cochlear damage in the form of hearing loss and tinnitus. Vancomycin (Vancocin, Vancoled), can also cause cochleotoxic damage, many times permanent. Minocycline (Minocin, Vectrin), a tetracycline,

Table 34-3: Some Drugs Containing Quinines

Legatrin	Quin-260	Quin-Amino	Quinamm
Quindan	Quiphile	Q-Vel	quinidine gluconate (Duraquin, Quinaglute Duratabs, Quinate, Quinatime, Quin-Release)
hydroxy-chloroquine (plaquenil)	chloroquine (Aralen)	quinidine polygalac-turonate (Cardioquin)	quinidine sulfate (Apo-Quinidine, CinQuin, Novoquinidin, Quinidex Exentabs, Quinora, SK-Quinidine Sulfate)

Table 34-4: Aminoglycoside Antibiotics That Can Be Ototoxic

streptomycin	tobramycin (Nebcin, Tobrex)	amikacin (Amikin)
gentamicin Garamycin, Gentacidin, G-Mycin, Gentafair, Gentak, Jenamicin)	kanamycin (Anamid, Kantrex, Klebcil)	neomycin (Mycifradin, Myciguent)
netilmicin (Netromycin)	paromomycin (humatin)	dibekacin
framycetin	ribostamycin	sisomicin

causes temporary vestibular changes in 30 to 90 percent of those taking it.

Table 34-6, next page, lists potentially cochleotoxic chemicals. Of the chemicals in this table, manganese, mercury, and trichloroethylene have also been reported to be vestibulotoxic.

Table 34-7, next page, lists some of the substances that can contain one or more ototoxic chemicals.

Exposure to ototoxic chemicals may also occur during electroplating, shoe manufacturing, dry cleaning, cold vulcanization, electronic battery manufacture, and polyvinyl chloride manufacturing.

Table 34-5: Anti-Cancer Drugs That Can Cause Permanent Cochlear Damage

carmustine (BiCNU)	cisplatin (Platinol)	carboplatin (Paraplatin, CBDCA)
nitrogen mustard (chlorambucil, estramustine phosphate sodium, mechlorethamine HCl, mustine, melphalan, uracil mustard)	vincristine (LCR, Oncovin, VCR)	vinblastine (Velban, Velbe, VLB)
DFMO	bleomycin	actinomycin
misonidazole		

Table 34-6: Chemicals That Are Potentially Cochleotoxic

strychnine	styrene	gold
formaldehyde	mercury*	butyl nitrite
benzene vapors	manganese*	trichloro-ethylene*
toluene	lead	hexane
arsenic	tin aniline dyes	ergot
carbon disulfite	carbon monoxide	xylene
potassium bromate		

*also reported to be vestibulotoxic

Table 34-7: Some Substances That Can Contain One or More Ototoxic Chemicals

grease remover	spot remover	rug cleaner
paint	varnish	thinner
resin	insulation	room odorizer
glue	auto emissions	spray paint
organic solvent	insecticide	lacquer
adhesive	coverup fluid such	fungicide
wood preservative	as White-Out	

Steps you can take:

- If you regularly use any of the potentially ototoxic medications, discuss their use with your doctor.
- When you select an over-the-counter analgesic or fever reducer, acetominophen (Tylenol) would probably be the best choice.
- When you use household chemicals, particularly those mentioned above, do so in a well- ventilated area. (Open the windows or doors,

at least two, for cross-ventilation, and possibly supplement with a fan.)
• Avoid exposure to lead (found in dilapidated buildings, buildings from the 1950s or before under renovation, some water supplies, and from lead processing plants.)
• Don't drink large amounts of tonic water.
• Don't take any aminoglycoside antibiotics (Table 34-4) or vancomycin unless you have a serious infection that cannot be treated with anything else.

Ears and Eyes

Infection

The ear (both cochlear and vestibular areas) can be damaged by infection from virus or bacteria (including a head cold, flu, meningitis, swimmer's ear, or sore throat).
Steps you can take:
• Insert ear plugs when you swim.
• Keep immunizations up to date including MMR (mumps, measles, rubella), influenza (flu), and pneumonia.
• Seek treatment if you think you have a bacterial infection of the nose, throat, or ear.
• Wash your hands after being exposed to someone with a cold.
Your eyes can be damaged permanently by some infections, or they can be temporarily affected by other infections such as conjunctivitis.
Steps you can take:
• Seek treatment if your eyes become red, itch or burn, and have drainage, particularly if its color is green.
• Don't share makeup with other people, particularly if their eyes appear to be red or abnormal in any way.

Ears, Eyes, Brain

Drug Effects

The vestibular system and brain can be temporarily impaired by the use of alcohol and drugs such as the temporary vestibular symptom blockers, pain killers, muscle relaxants, tranquilizers, and some anesthetic agents (particularly during general anesthesia).

Steps you can take:

- Don't drink alcohol.
- If you take any of these problem drugs, be prepared to have balance problems.
- If you use any of these drugs, take care when walking.
- If you use any of these drugs, don't drive or do anything requiring good coordination or balance.
- Plan to have extra help moving about if you are taking pain killers or undergoing general anesthesia.
- Avoid throw rugs and cluttered floors.

Vision can be impaired by temporary vestibular symptom blockers if they cause dilation. Dilation will cause blurred vision which, at times, can be extreme.

Steps you can take:

- If you have blurred vision, don't drive.
- Be careful when walking, even at home.

Trauma

Trauma can injure the ear, eyes, and brain, sometimes all three at the same time. Some examples are foreign object insertion (cotton swab such as Q-Tip, bobby pin, etc.) into the ear, foreign object in the eye, or a blow to the head, ear, or eye.

Steps you can take:

- Insert nothing into the ear canal (except ear plugs) including cotton swabs such as Q-Tips. (If itching or wax are a problem, consult your M.D.)
- Wear a helmet when bicycling, rollerblading, riding a motorcycle, and during any other activity that can result in a head injury.
- Use a seat belt when you travel in cars and airplanes.
- Avoid activities that create a high chance of head or ear trauma.
- Wear eye goggles when you work with drills, saws, and other tools that can send slivers of foreign objects or sawdust into the air, when you play racquetball, ride a bike or motorcycle, rollerblade in windy conditions, and when you swim.
- Use eye glasses with UV protection when you are outside, particularly in the sun.
- Do not stare at the sun, such as during an eclipse, or at halogen light bulbs.
- Avoid or take great care around firecrackers.

Vision

Vision is one of the three systems we use to maintain good balance function. People with vestibular problems can come to depend heavily upon vision to maintain balance. A decrease in vision can easily result in more symptoms, such as feeling unsteady, and decreased balance ability.

Vision can be impaired by trauma (discussed above), ultraviolet light, disease (glaucoma, diabetes mellitus), the natural changes responsible for nearsightedness and farsightedness, poor lighting conditions, wearing glasses with the wrong prescription, and wearing glasses with a new prescription strength.

Steps you can take:

• Have a yearly vision exam if you wear glasses or are over 40.

• Have a yearly glaucoma check if you are 40 or over.

• When planning a trip to the ophthalmologist or optometrist, take along an adult who can drive and act as a physical support in case your pupils are dilated and you have balance difficulties.

• Be careful when first wearing glasses with a new prescription. Your balance may become more impaired until you adjust.

• Install or have someone else install adequate lighting in your home and its entrances. Use more lighting as you age.

• Be careful when peeling onions or when engaged in any other activity that can reduce your vision because of blinking or tear production.

• Keep a flashlight handy when you are away from home in the dark.

• Keep supplies for emergency lighting on hand such as a flashlight with charged batteries, candles, a camping lantern, and battery-powered emergency lighting.

Proprioception

We also depend on proprioception for balance. Individuals with a vestibular disorder can come to depend heavily upon proprioception to maintain balance. Because of this, damage or decreased proprioceptive function can have a large impact.

Proprioception can be damaged by trauma (to the arms and legs or the nervous system) and diseases such as diabetes mellitus. Temporary problems can occur when you move about in windy conditions, walk on soft surfaces such as a padded rug or sand or mud, or if circulation is slowed to one of your limbs.

Steps you can take:

- Do not walk barefoot on a hot or potentially hot surface or in a place where your feet can be damaged by stepping on glass, stones, etc.
- Maintain ideal weight.
- If you have diabetes, work closely with your doctor on blood sugar control.
- Avoid leg crossing while you sit.
- Don't sit with your legs "scrunched up" under your bottom.
- If one of your legs is found to be "sleeping," allow feeling to return before trying to walk.

Alertness

Adequate alertness is needed for proper balance. Alertness can be temporarily reduced by drugs, alcohol, or fatigue. It can also be reduced if the brain is damaged by disease or trauma.

Steps you can take:

- Get enough sleep each night.
- Be careful when you become greatly fatigued.

Muscle Strength

Muscle strength is another ingredient for balance. It can be temporarily reduced by decreased or inadequate use and permanently impaired through disease or trauma. The muscles can also be affected by sudden overuse and the stiffening this causes.

Steps you can take:

- Do not overexercise.
- Exercise according to your abilities, your physical shape, and your physician's directions.

Joint Flexibility

Joint flexibility can be temporarily impaired by under- or overuse and permanently affected by the presence of disease (such as arthritis) or trauma.

Steps you can take:

- Do not overexercise.
- If you are accustomed to exercising, include types that put the joints through all their movements.

References

_____. *The Physician's Desk Reference.* Oradell, N.J.: Medical Economics, 1994.

_____. U.S. Preventive Services Task Force. *Guide to Clinical Protective Services: An Assessment of the Effectiveness of 169 Interventions.* Baltimore: Williams and Wilkins, 1989.

Black, F.O., and Pesznecker, S.C. "Vestibular Ototoxicity: Clinical Considerations." *Otolaryngology Clinics of North America,* 26:713-736, 1993.

Boettcher, F.A., and Salvi, R.J. "Salicylate Ototoxicity: Review and Synthesis." *American Journal of Otolaryngology,* 12:33-47, 1991.

Dobie, R.A. "Prevention of Noise-Induced Hearing Loss." *Archives of Otolaryngology-Head and Neck Surgery,* 121:385-391, 1995.

Haye, A.W. *Toxicology of the Eye, Ear, and Other Special Senses.* New York: Raven Press, 1985.

Jung, T.T., Rhee, C.K., Lee, C.S., Park, Y.S., and Choi, D.C. "Ototoxicity of Salicylate, Nonsteroidal Anti-Inflammatory Drugs, and Quinine." *Otolaryngology Clinics of North America,* 26:791-807, 1993.

Kennie, D.C. *Preventive Care for Elderly People.* Cambridge: Cambridge University Press, 1993.

McCombe, A.W., Binnington, J., Davis, A., and Spencer, H. "Hearing Loss and Motorcyclists." *Journal of Laryngology and Otology,* 109:599-604, 1995.

Pollock, K., and Pebworth, D. "Protect Yourself from Noise-Induced Hearing Loss. *Notes* (Acoustic Neuroma Association), 53:1-3, 1995.

Ryback, L.P. "Hearing: The Effects of Chemicals." *Otolaryngology— Head and Neck Surgery,* 106:677-685, 1992.

Sanford, J.P. *Guide to Antimicrobial Therapy.* Dallas, Tex.: Antimicrobial Therapy, Inc., 1993.

Schweitzer, V.G. "Ototoxicity of Chemotherapeutic Agents." *Otolaryngologic Clinics of North America,* 26:759-783, 1993.

Tianwu, H., Watanabe, M., Shimizu, K., Takada, S., and Mizukoshi, K. "Effect of Alcohol Ingestion on Vestibular Function in Postural Control." *Acta Otolaryngologica, Supplement,* 519: 127-131, 1995.

Whitener, C.J., and Parker, J.E. "Erythromycin Ototoxicity: A Call to Heighten Recognition." *Southern Medical Journal,* 84:1214-1216, 1991.

Chapter 35

Research

B ecause no cure exists for Meniere's disease and so little is known about it, research offers possibilities for success. For example, research might reveal information about inner ear changes caused by Meniere's disease, basic ear function and structure, normal development and aging, eye control, immune function, nerve signal transmission chemicals, and hair cell regeneration. Such information might lead to better diagnosis and treatment.

Research is carried out in the U.S. and worldwide by many people. Projects are done in universities, hospitals, institutes, and doctors' offices by Ph.D.s, M.D.s, audiologists, biomedical engineers, physical therapists, and others. Research money comes from multiple sources.

Who Is in Charge?

"Nobody," is the short answer to the question of who's in charge of Meniere's research. There is no coordinated "war on Meniere's disease" and no central person or organization giving the marching orders. However, those handling the research money have a great deal of influence over what is studied.

Organizations such as the U.S. Federal government or the Deafness Research Foundation, which fund research by competition for grants, generally have long-term goals or objectives formulated by groups of research scientists. Researchers, guided by the goals and findings of previous research, devise projects and do their best to write compelling research proposals. Funding organizations usually choose projects on the basis of how well they will help meet the organizations' goals, how they are designed, and which have the best chance of collecting valuable data.

Scientists are said to compete for funds, and this is accurate. Winners get research money, and others do not.

Who Pays?

A large number of funding sources, both public and private, contribute to Meniere's research. At the 1997 winter meeting of the

Association for Research in Otolaryngology, representatives from more than 60 organizations from 17 countries listed more than a thousand ongoing research projects related to otolaryngology. Of course, only some of those were related to Meniere's disease.

Non-governmental sources of funds include nonprofit organizations like the Deafness Research Foundation, the American Tinnitus Association, the American Otological Society, and the National Organization for Hearing Research. Corporations such as pharmaceutical and medical equipment companies also at times support research involving their products. In addition, physicians or physician groups sometimes set up nonprofit foundations to raise money for their own research.

United States

Below are descriptions of a few, but not all, sources of Meniere's research funds in the U.S. The Federal government is the largest source of these funds. Branches of this government that conduct Meniere's research include the National Institutes of Health (NIH), the National Science Foundation (NSF), the National Aeronautics and Space Administration (NASA), the Office of Naval Research (ONR), the Department of Veterans Affairs (VA), the Department of Education, and the U.S. Army.

The NIH

The U.S. National Institutes of Health (NIH), headquartered in Bethesda, Maryland, is the largest Federal agency for biomedical research. In 1996, the total budget for research activities by the NIH was $12 billion (for all research activities, not for Meniere's disease). The total budget for the NIH and other Federal agencies is set by the U.S. Congress.

The NIH is one of eight agencies of the Public Health Service within the U.S. Department of Health and Human Services.

The mission of the NIH is "to uncover new knowledge that will lead to better health for everyone." It carries out this mission by awarding money for research projects, financing science training by supporting science students, providing funds for beginning researchers, and funding research training centers. Only a small amount of this work is conducted at its Maryland home; the rest is done in locations throughout the country.

The NIH is divided into 18 different institutes including deafness and other communication disorders (NIDCD), cancer, eye, genome, aging, dental, heart/lung/blood, alcohol abuse/alcoholism, allergy/infectious diseases, arthritis/musculoskeletal/skin diseases, child health/human development, drug abuse, diabetes/digestive/kidney, environmental health sciences, general medical sciences, mental health, neurological disorders/stroke, and nursing research.

The institute overseeing the inner ear is the National Institute for Deafness and Other Communication Disorders (NIDCD) headed by James. F. Battey, Jr., M.D., Ph.D.

The NIDCD

The NIDCD is the National Institute on Deafness and Other Communication Disorders. The functions included within this branch of the National Institutes of Health (NIH) are hearing, balance, smell, taste, language, voice, and speech.

During fiscal year 1994, 4 percent of the NIDCD budget went for the study of balance and 57 percent for hearing. During fiscal year 1995, 7 percent ($9.1 million) of the NIDCD budget went for the study of balance and 53 percent for hearing. (The other funding included 10 percent for smell, 5 percent for taste, 5 percent for voice, 9 percent for speech, and 11 percent for language.) The fiscal year 1997 appropriation (budget amount) from Congress is for $188 million, a 6.8 percent ($12 million) increase over fiscal year 1996.

Because vestibular function is so important and because vestibular disturbances can cause problems in many areas of the body, other institutes also fund research related to balance. In 1995, the National Eye Institute spent $4.7 million, NASA $4.4 million, and the National Institute on Aging $2.5 million. These are funds spent on balance research, not just Meniere's disease.

NIDCD goals for balance are developed and published as the National Strategic Research Plan for balance every few years. This plan describes progress in balance research and outlines areas of need. The most recent plan was written for 1994-1995. Areas identified for further study included ion transport, neurotransmitters, normal development, aging, hair cell regeneration, genetics, gaze control, posture control, spatial orientation, diagnostic testing, immune reactions/diseases, autonomic nervous system control, physical therapy, aminoglycoside destruction procedures, monitoring during inner ear surgeries, a better animal model to study, and fluid transport in epithelial tissues other than the ear.

To partially fulfill its goals, the NIDCD funds six large ongoing projects: the national multipurpose research and training center for balance at the University of California at Los Angeles (UCLA), the national multipurpose research and training center for hearing and balance at Johns Hopkins University, the national research and training center for childhood deafness at the Boys Town National Research Hospital, the NIDCD Information Clearinghouse for the dispersal of information to the public, the National Temporal Bone, Hearing and Balance Pathology Resource Registry to promote temporal bone donation and research, and the NIDCD/NASA multi-institutional center for vestibular research at the Robert S. Dow Neurological Sciences Institute in Portland and Northwestern University in Chicago. The NIDCD is also funding 15 studies in fiscal year 1997 that may provide information of importance for Meniere's disease. (See "U.S. Research Projects" later in this chapter.)

The NSF

Established by the National Science Foundation Act of 1950, the NSF is an independent agency of the U.S. Federal government. Its mission is to promote the progress of science; to advance the national health, prosperity, and welfare; and to secure the national defense. Its 1996 budget was $3.3 billion given to 20,000 research and education projects in science and engineering.

The Deafness Research Foundation

The Deafness Research Foundation (DRF) was founded in 1958 by Collette Ramsey-Baher. It is the nation's largest voluntary health organization entirely committed to public awareness and support for basic and clinical research into deafness and other serious ear disorders. In 1995, the DRF awarded $900,000 to fund 54 different projects. It awards competitive grants and monies to help promising students and doctors-in-training prepare for a career in research. The DRF depends upon contributions from citizens and corporations.

How to Encourage Research

Here are ways to encourage Meniere's research:

• Give money to organizations that fund research. (See Chapter 39, "Where to Get More Information.")

• In the U.S., help keep NIH funding at present levels or above by writing to your U.S. Representative and U.S. Senators.

• In the U.S., help keep National Science Foundation funding at present levels or above by writing to your U.S. Representative and U.S. Senators.

• In the U.S., sign up with the Temporal Bone Registry to donate your own temporal bones to science for possible study after you die.

• In other countries, call or write your own national Meniere's organization. Its representatives should be able to give you information specific to your country. Check for the names and addresses of some of these organizations in Chapter 39, "Where to Get More Information."

- If you want to make a contribution to an organization outside your country, remember to do it in the currency of the country you are sending it to.

Why Stay Hopeful About Research?

Because many bright, dedicated people worldwide are working to solve vestibular problems, you can remain hopeful that breakthroughs will occur during your lifetime.

Not only are scientists working on Meniere's disease, but they are also working on related areas such as hearing, space travel, flight medicine, alternative medicine, radiology, drug therapy, and genetics. These kinds of research, funded by many different organizations, may contribute to the understanding of the inner ear and Meniere's disease. It is not unusual for a breakthrough in one area to benefit others, a kind of scientific trickle-down.

U.S. Research Projects

Below are descriptions of some, but not all, ongoing research projects in the U.S. related to Meniere's disease. All of the quoted material comes from Computer Retrieval of Information on Scientific Projects (CRISP) documents of the National Institutes of Health. (See "References" at the end of this chapter.)

1997 NIDCD Research

- *Control Mechanisms in Sensory and Communication Disorders: Virus Specific IgE Mediated Immune Response and Meniere's Disease.*—Emanuel Calenoff, Northwestern University Medical School, Chicago, Ill.

  "Immunoglobulin E (IgE)—mediated immune reactivity may be targeted against latent herpes-family viruses located within the inner ear. Our preliminary studies, measuring herpes virus-specific IgE in the sera of Meniere's patients, suggest that most patients with Meniere's disease possess such reactivity. Most control subjects do not. The recurrent and reversible Meniere's symptoms: episodic vertigo, fluctuating hearing loss, tinnitus, and fullness, could all be caused by a latent IgE-mediated inflammatory response.

  "The specific aims of this research proposal are: 1) To examine the serum of patients with Meniere's disease for the presence of IgE that has specific reactivity to proteins of viruses that are known to be associated with latent viral infections, specifically herpes simplex type 1 and 2, Epstein-Barr virus, cytomegalovirus and/or varicella-zoster virus; and to determine whether patients with Meniere's disease are significantly different than the general population in the presence of IgE that is specific to those viruses. 2) To identify and define the principle proteins in these viruses to which IgE reacts."

• *Electron Microscopy of the Inner Ear*—Robert S. Kimura, Massachusetts Eye and Ear Infirmary, Boston, Mass.

"Our objective is to find the cause of and a cure for Meniere's disease by developing an animal model and using such a model for treatment.

"In the current animal model, the endolymphatic duct is tied off to create endolymphatic hydrops, but this method does not seem to cause episodic vertigo. This research will be exploring other ways to create the endolymphatic hydrops with vertigo such as applying pressure to the middle ear. Once endolymphatic hydrops with episodic vertigo can be created, more effective treatments may be found."

• *Electron Microscopy of the Human Inner Ear*—Joseph Nadol, Massachusetts Eye and Ear Infirmary, Boston, Mass.

"Histologic study at the level of light and electron microscopy of the normal and pathologic human inner ear and spiral ganglion is proposed."

(This study involves basic research to further understand the structure of the human inner ear on a microscopic level.)

• *Integrated Center for In Vivo Microscopy: MR Microscopy of Endolymphatic Hydrops*—Miriam Henson, Duke University Medical Center, Durham, N.C.

"Endolymphatic hydrops is an enlargement of the scala media which occurs in various pathological conditions, e.g. Meniere's disease. Study of hydrops is highly clinically relevant in that it is one of the most common causes of hearing impairment in humans. The purpose of the present research is to follow the normal progression of endolymphatic hydrops as it occurs in the guinea pig and/or gerbil. To date, this has not been possible because of the lack of a noninvasive technique for assessing the dimensions of the scala media. The guinea pig is currently an accepted model of endolymphatic hydrops and it can be artificially created by occluding the endolymphatic duct; preliminary data obtained with the mustached bat cochlea *ex vivo* has shown the feasibility of such a study. After the normal sequence of development of hydrops is described, then various manipulations, i.e., different drugs without serious side effects to the animals, can be used to try to alleviate this condition. Since the final goal of this research is to observe the *in vivo* progression of endolymphatic hydrops, the smaller gerbil may be the animal of choice."

In depth (*in vivo*): Study *in vivo* refers to the study of something within a living creature rather than, say, in a test tube.

• *Inner Ear Fluid Interactions*—Alec N. Salt, Washington University, St. Louis
"The goal of this proposal is to establish how endolymph composition and volume are regulated. Lack of knowledge in this area severely limits our understanding of disease processes of the inner ear, such as Meniere's disease and perilymph fistula.
"Only by understanding the relationships between mechanical, chemical and physiological processes can we hope to understand how endolymph volume is regulated and how disturbances of volume can be treated in patients."

• *Cochlear and Vestibular Ion Transport*—Daniel C. Marcus, Boys Town National Research Hospital, Omaha, Neb.
"Meniere's disease is one of the pathological entities characterized by endolymphatic hydrops of the cochlear and vestibular labyrinths. Hydrops can result from an alteration of ion transport. . . ."

In depth (ions): When chemicals called electrolytes are placed into a fluid, their constituent parts will have either a positive or a negative charge. These charged parts are called ions.

• *Inner Ear Ion Transport Mechanisms*—Bradley A. Shulte, Medical University of South Carolina
". . . little is yet known about the specific cellular and molecular mechanisms that produce the unique ion and electrical gradients in the inner ear. Such knowledge is essential because imbalances in ionic or electrical gradients are involved in hearing losses associated with metabolic disorders, ischemic events, Meniere's disease, and aging. It also is probable that alterations in cellular ion homeostasis promote the damage to hair cells induced by noise and ototoxic drugs."

• *Biomedical Simulations Resource: Modeling of Vestibulo-Ocular Reflex as an Adaptive Control System*—Dennis P. O'Leary, University of Southern California, Los Angeles, Calif.
"This project studies the dynamics of the VOR as an adaptive control system during the compensation periods of selected patients and the normal subjects undergoing high-frequency testing."

- *Research and Training Center in Hearing and Balance: Vestibular Reflex Adaptation—Physical Rehabilitation/Surgical Interventions* —David S. Zee, Johns Hopkins School of Medicine, Baltimore, Md. "Patients who undergo acute unilateral vestibular deafferentation (UVD), as a surgical intervention for acoustic neuroma or Meniere's disease, suffer from a variety of vestibular, oculomotor, and postural disorders. This leads to problems of postural stability, disorientation, dizziness, and blurred vision during head motion. We propose a series of studies designed to enhance our knowledge of the process of compensation to UVD."
- *Molecular Basis of Vestibular Efferent Function*—Phillip A. Wackym, Mount Sinai School of Medicine, New York, N.Y.
  "The long term objective of this research is to understand the projection of the vestibular efferent neurons to the vestibular periphery in the context of the fundamental molecular sensory organization of the receptor and the vestibular primary afferents.
  "This research will help our understanding of outgoing and incoming vestibular nerve messages during vestibular compensation, after a vestibular injury, and with specific vestibular disorders like Meniere's disease. It may also lead to improvements in drug treatments for these disorders."
- *Cochlear Blood Flow and Neuropeptides*—Alfred L. Nuttall, Oregon Health Sciences University, Portland, Ore.
  "This proposal seeks to define the mechanisms of cochlear blood flow."
- *Vestibular Reflex Recovery After Neurotological Surgery*—Stephen P. Cass, Eye and Ear Institute of Pittsburgh, Pa.
  "The objective of the proposed research is to improve the treatment of patients with balance disorders by providing new information about the response of the vestibular system to neurotological surgery."
- *Loudness Summation, Lateralization, and Fusion*—Bertram Scharf, Northeastern University, Boston, Mass.
  "The other broad goal of this proposal is to identify the functions of the olivocochlear bundle in human hearing. This bundle of some 900 nerve fibers sends signals from the brain to the receptors in the inner ear. To determine how these fibers affect hearing, patients who have had their vestibular nerve cut to relieve intractable vertigo, usually caused by Meniere's disease, will be studied."
- *Basic and Clinical Studies of the Auditory System: Inner Ear—Ion Homeostasis in the Sensory Epithelium*—Edmund Mroz, Massachusetts Eye and Ear Infirmary, Boston, Mass.
  "The link between homeostasis and signal processing may have important pathophysiologic implications. Altered intracellular ionic composition may lead to changes, both reversible and irre-

versible, in cells. Thus they may play critical roles in either short- or long-term hearing losses observed in many conditions such as Meniere's disease, overstimulation, or ototoxicity."

(This study will look at the chemicals in endolymph and perilymph because their imbalance may cause the hearing loss found in Meniere's disease.)

National Science Foundation (Vestibular Projects)

- *NASA Neurolab: Development of Vestibular Organs in Microgravity*—Micheal Wiederhof, University of Texas Health Sciences Center, San Antonio, Tex.
- *Visual Control of Posture Within the Normal Range of Motion*— Thomas Stoffregen, University of Cincinnati, Ohio
- *Acquisition of Transmission Electron Microscope for Biological Sciences*—Robert S. Hikida, Ohio University
- *Computational Modeling of the Rodent Head Direction Systems*, David S. Touretzky, Carnegie Mellon University, Pittsburgh, Pa.

The House Ear Institute

This organization includes a branch of the National Temporal Bone Registry and is currently researching the endolymphatic sac, effectiveness of allergy treatment on Meniere's disease, autoimmune hearing loss, and the use of ginkgo biloba extract to treat tinnitus. The institute is also funding a study by Gwen Morse, R.N., Ph.D., on the relationship between Meniere's disease and the menstrual cycle.

The American Nurses' Foundation

This organization is funding a second study by Gwen Morse, R.N., Ph.D., on Meniere's disease and the menstrual cycle.

John's Hopkins University School of Medicine

Researchers at the laboratory of vestibular neurophysiology at Johns Hopkins are studying the organization and control of vestibular reflexes. They are also investigating the physiological processes involved in compensation for a unilateral vestibular injury.

Massachusetts Eye and Ear Infirmary

In addition to carrying out the electron microscopy and ion

264 ❖ Meniere's Disease—What You Need to Know

homeostasis studies cited earlier, health professionals at the Massachusetts Eye and Ear Infirmary oversee the work of the National Temporal Bone Bank, which is based there. They are also conducting research on immune-mediated Meniere's disease.

Meniere's Research Elsewhere

Below are descriptions of some, but not all, ongoing Meniere's-related research projects in countries other than the U.S.

University of Sussex, U.K.

At the University of Sussex, basic hearing research is carried out by about 25 people in three groups. Science students, doctors-in-training, scientists-in-training, and experienced scientists are involved. Funding comes from a number of sources including the Wolfson Foundation, Hearing Research Trust, Royal Society, a European Laboratory Network grant, the European Science Foundation, and Smith-Kline.

Southampton University Hospital, U.K.

In the non-invasive pressure assessment unit of Southampton University, scientists are studying the pressure of inner ear fluids.

MRC Institute of Hearing Research, University of Nottingham, U.K.

The MRC Institute is conducting research on hearing and virtual reality applications.

Institute of Biomedical Engineering, Bio-medical Acoustics Group, University of Toronto, Canada

The Biomedical Acoustics Group researches the auditory processes of living creatures and studies the scientific and engineering aspects of acoustics and hearing.

References

_____. *Annual Report—1995*. Bethesda, Md.: National Institute on Deafness and Other Communication Disorders (NIDCD).

_____. *National Strategic Research Plan, 1994-1995: Language and Language Impairments, Balance and Balance Disorders, Voice and Voice Disorders* (NIH Publication No. 96-3217). Bethesda, Md.: National Institute on Deafness and Other Communication Disorders (NIDCD).

National Institutes of Health. "Notice Concerning the CRISP System on Gopher," http://www.nih.gov/grants/award/gophercrisp.htm. July 15, 1997.

Snow, J.B. "News from the National Institute on Deafness and Other Communication Disorders." *American Journal of Otology,* 15(2):132-136, 1996.

Snow, J.B. "News from the National Institute on Deafness and Other Communication Disorders." *American Journal of Otology,* 18(3): 285-287, 1997.

Chapter 36

Temporal Bone Research and Donation

T he temporal bone is a part of the skull that houses the outer,
middle, and inner ears. The inner ear contains the organs of
hearing (cochlea) and balance (semicircular canals and
otoliths). The cochlear and the vestibular nerves convey information
from the inner ear to the brain regarding hearing and balance respec-
tively.

The inner ear (also known as the labyrinth) is not accessible for
direct examination and study during life. One reason is that it is deep
seated within the temporal bone and therefore cannot be examined.
A surgical biopsy of the inner ear is impractical since it would result
in severe hearing loss or balance disturbance. Hence, information
about disorders affecting the inner ear is obtained indirectly by means
of hearing tests (e.g., audiograms), balance tests (e.g., ENG) and by
imaging studies (e.g., CT and MRI scans). At present, imaging does
not have sufficient resolution to allow for detailed assessment of the
fine structural details of the inner ear.

How Is It Studied?

One of the best ways to study the inner ear is to examine the temporal bone after death. Such bones are obtained from people who have
donated or pledged their temporal bones for research after their death. A

*This chapter was contributed to this book by Saumil N. Merchant,
M.D., of the Harvard Medical School and Massachusetts Eye and Ear
Infirmary and the NIDCD National Temporal Bone, Hearing and
Balance Pathology Resource Registry, both in Boston, Massachusetts,
and by Sumiko M. Goldbaum, B.S., of the NIDCD National Temporal
Bone, Hearing and Balance Pathology Resource Registry, Boston,
Massachusetts.*

268 ❖ Meniere's Disease—What You Need to Know

small part of the temporal bone (only the part containing the middle and inner ears) is surgically removed soon after death. This removal does not affect the appearance of the donor's outer ear, face, or head. The temporal bone is then prepared for a variety of research techniques.

The standard technique consists of light microscopy, which involves the following steps: fixing the temporal bone in formalin to preserve the various delicate structures of the inner ear, decalcifying the bone to soften it, infiltrating the bone with a substance like celloidin so that it can be sectioned, sectioning or slicing the bone, and finally, staining it with haematoxylin and eosin. Each temporal bone usually yields 400 to 500 serial sections, of which about 40 are selected and stained for study. The other non-stained sections are saved for future use. This technique of preparation for light microscopy needs special equipment and expertise, is time consuming, tedious, and expensive. For example, it takes approximately two years and $1,000 to $2,000 per bone. However, such study is well worth the time and the expense because it can yield a tremendous amount of useful information that cannot be obtained in any other way. There are only a handful of laboratories in the United States and in the world which perform such temporal bone research.

Besides standard light microscopy, a variety of newer research techniques have been developed in the past several years that have enhanced the value of this type of research. These newer techniques include electron microscopy, immuno-staining, computer-aided reconstruction, and procedures that allow identification of defects at a molecular level (molecular biology). The newer techniques hold promise in providing clues and answers to many of the mysteries of Meniere's disease and of other disorders affecting the inner ear.

Information from Temporal Bone Research

Studies have shown that the following changes can occur within the inner ears in Meniere's disease.

Endolymphatic Hydrops

Endolymphatic hydrops refers to distention or swelling of the membranous labyrinth (the compartment containing endolymph). Endolymphatic hydrops is a consistent finding in Meniere's disease. The hydrops mainly involves the cochlear duct and saccule but can also involve the utricle and semicircular canals. In some cases, the hydrops is severe, and it results in distortion and collapse of the walls of the membranous labyrinth. Figure 36-1 shows a section through a

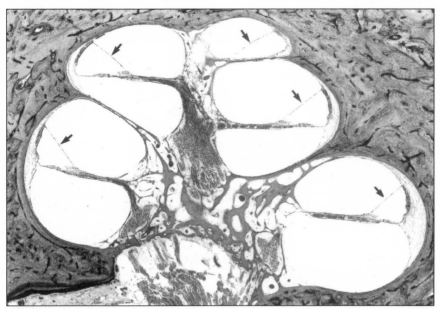

Figure 36-1: Normal cochlea. This is a cross-section of a cochlea from a 71-year-old man. Reissner's membrane, indicated by arrows, is in the normal position. For clarity, the actual cochlea has been magnified by a factor of 19.

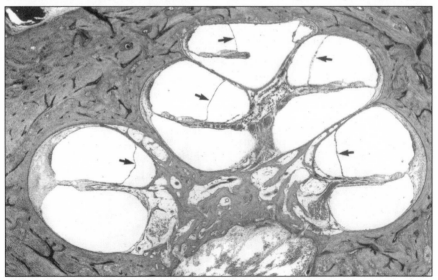

Figure 36-2: Cochlea showing endolymphatic hydrops. This is a cross-section of a cochlea from a 65-year-old woman with Meniere's disease. Endolymphatic hydrops is manifested by distention of Reissner's membrane, indicated by arrows. For clarity, the actual cochlea has been magnified by a factor of 18. (These two photos courtesy of the Otopathology Laboratory at the Massachusetts Eye and Ear Infirmary, Boston, Massachusetts.)

normal cochlea, while Figure 36-2 is that from a cochlea with Meniere's disease showing hydrops.

Sensory and Neural Lesions

In most cases of Meniere's disease, light microscopy of temporal bone sections has shown that the sensory hair cells and neurons within the cochlea and the vestibular system are present in normal numbers. Because of this finding, it has been proposed that the endolymphatic hydrops is somehow responsible for the episodic vertigo and fluctuating hearing loss.

In the later stages of Meniere's disease, the hearing loss becomes non-fluctuant and there is often loss of word recognition (speech discrimination) ability. Even though the hair cells and neurons are present in normal numbers, studies have shown a striking and significant reduction in the number of nerve endings and synapses. This finding can explain the occurrence of permanent hearing loss, especially the poor word recognition ability.

Vestibular Fibrosis

Proliferation of fibrous tissue can occur within the vestibule of the inner ear that results in the formation of a band that connects the stapes footplate to the utricle or saccule. This change is called vestibular fibrosis, and it may account for a positive Hennebert's sign (a positive fistula sign without a fistula) which is observed in about 30 percent of patients with Meniere's disease.

Endolymphatic Sac Abnormalities

Much attention has focused on the endolymphatic sac and its relationship to the production of endolymphatic hydrops. Some investigators have found abnormalities in the sac, which has led them to believe that dysfunction of the sac leads to production of hydrops. On the other hand, other investigators have not been able to corroborate the observed abnormalities within the sac.

What Areas Need Further Research?

Currently, much more research is needed in the area of pathology and pathophysiology of Meniere's disease. For example, even though it is currently believed by most that endolymphatic hydrops produces the clinical symptoms and signs of Meniere's disease, this belief has not been proven beyond doubt. Establishing the precise relationship between hydrops and symptoms and signs is critical to our understanding of the disease and also critical to developing ways to treat it as well as control it.

Meniere's disease is a relatively common disorder and it has been estimated that approximately 100,000 cases of Meniere's disease are treated every year in just the United States. Yet, there have been only about 100 temporal bone cases of Meniere's disease described in the word literature to date and many of these cases lack good clinical documentation of symptoms, signs and test findings. Furthermore, the number of cases in which electron microscopy studies have been done is less than 10. Thus, there is a great need for the study of many more well-documented cases with accompanying medical histories and audiometric and vestibular test results in order to enable scientists and researchers to fully understand the spectrum of pathologic changes in this condition. To date, there are still no well-documented temporal bone reports of the pathologic changes in the inner ear in Lermoyez's syndrome, in Tumarkin's drop attack, in "cochlear" Meniere's disease, and in "vestibular" Meniere's disease. There is also little published temporal bone information about the efficacy of various medical and surgical procedures for Meniere's disease, and yet hundreds of these operations are performed annually in the United States alone.

Temporal bone research is critical in order to enable us to understand the pathophysiology of Meniere's disease. Once this is accomplished, it will enable us to devise medical and other therapies in order to prevent the progression of hearing loss once Meniere's disease has been established and also to prevent the occurrence of vertigo. It may also be possible to prevent the disease from affecting the opposite ear.

Donating Your Temporal Bones

Persons affected by Meniere's disease can contribute to advances in understanding and treating it by pledging to donate their temporal bones for research purposes after death. Such research will make it possible to provide others with the gift of balance and hearing in the future. People who wish to donate their temporal bones can do so by contacting the NIDCD National Temporal Bone Registry and enrolling in its National Temporal Bone Donor Program. This is described later. Those who donate their temporal bones should also consider donating the brain stem, where some of the brain pathways for balance and hearing are located.

National Temporal Bone Registry

The NIDCD National Temporal Bone, Hearing and Balance Pathology Resource Registry is a nonprofit organization. It was established in 1992 by the National Institute on Deafness and Other Communication Disorders (NIDCD) of the National Institutes of Health, the Federal government's focal point for biomedical and behavioral research on hearing and balance. The Registry continues and expands on the activities of the former National Temporal Bone Banks Program, which was created in 1960 to encourage temporal bone donation. The Registry serves both the public and the scientific community by providing the following resources and services:

- enrollment of temporal bone donors
- 24-hour nationwide network to collect temporal bones after a donor's death
- computerized database of all human temporal bone collections in the United States
- dissemination of public information on temporal bone donation
- publication of a semi-annual newsletter, *The Registry*
- conservation of existing human temporal bone collections
- professional educational activities to teach physicians and scientists about temporal bone research

The Registry's national office is located at the Massachusetts Eye and Ear Infirmary in Boston, Massachusetts. The Registry works closely with all of the nation's 26 temporal bone research laboratories listed below:

Armed Forces Institute of Pathology/Walter Reed Army Medical Center, Washington, D.C.

Baylor College of Medicine, Houston, Texas

Bowman Gray School of Medicine, Winston-Salem, North Carolina

Columbia–Presbyterian Medical Center, New York, New York

Goodhill Ear Center-UCLA School of Medicine, Los Angeles, California

Henry Ford Hospital, Detroit, Michigan

House Ear Institute, Los Angeles, California

J. Hillis Miller Health Center, Gainesville, Florida

Kresge Hearing Research Institute-University of Michigan, Ann Arbor, Michigan

Massachusetts Eye and Ear Infirmary, Boston, Massachusetts

Mt. Sinai School of Medicine, New York, New York

New England Medical Center Hospitals, Boston, Massachusetts

New York University, New York, New York

Northwestern University Medical School, Chicago, Illinois
Otological Research Laboratories, Columbus, Ohio
Shea Clinic Foundation, Memphis, Tennessee
SUNY Health Science Center, Syracuse, New York
The Eye and Ear Institute of Pittsburgh, Pittsburgh, Pennsylvania
The Johns Hopkins University, Baltimore, Maryland
The University of Iowa Hospitals and Clinics, Iowa City, Iowa
University of Chicago, Chicago, Illinois
University of Colorado Health Science Center, Denver, Colorado
University of Minnesota, Minneapolis, Minnesota
University of Oklahoma Health Sciences Center, Oklahoma City, Oklahoma
University of Texas Southwestern Medical Center, Dallas, Texas
University of Wisconsin Hospital, Madison, Wisconsin

Questions About Donation

Here are common questions and their answers regarding temporal bone donations. If you have other questions, please contact the Temporal Bone Registry for further information.

Is there an age restriction?

No. No one is too young or too old to be a donor. Age does not affect the scientific value of your temporal bones.

Does removal of the temporal bones change the donor's appearance?

No. Removal of the temporal bones (and brain stem) does not change the appearance of the head, face, or outer ear. So, it does not affect funeral or burial arrangements, including an open casket.

Is there a cost to the donor's family or estate?

No. The medical professionals who remove the temporal bones donate their time or are paid by the laboratory receiving the temporal bones.

Is an autopsy necessary?

The consent form in your temporal bone donor packet gives permission for a limited autopsy for temporal bone (and related brain tissue) removal. In special circumstances, temporal bones may be removed without an autopsy.

Can I donate my body to science for anatomical study and also donate my temporal bones?

It depends. The policies of donor programs for anatomical study vary. Discuss this with your local body donor program to determine whether it is possible to donate to one or both programs.

Can I donate other organs for transplantation as well as my temporal bones?

Yes. The removal of your temporal bones would simply be delayed a few hours so that transplantable organs can be removed first.

What is the role of my next of kin?

In most states, the next of kin makes the final decision about organ or body donations. Inform them and your doctors of your wish to be a temporal bone donor. Be sure that they understand that their cooperation is needed.

How to Enroll as a Donor

- Contact the Registry by calling its 24-hour toll-free number (800) 822-1327 (voice) or (617) 573-3888 (TTY) or by e-mail at tbregistry@meei.harvard.edu. The Registry will send you a donor enrollment packet, which includes a medical history questionnaire and a donation and consent form.

- Return the completed forms and the Registry will send you a wallet-size Donor Card that states you are a temporal bone donor. The card also states that at the time of your death, your doctor or next of kin should call the Registry day or night at (800) 822-1327. The Registry will then coordinate the removal of your temporal bones.

- The Registry keeps a computerized record of all donations. It will also forward a copy of your pledge to the collaborating laboratory that is located nearest to you. This laboratory will eventually receive your temporal bones for study.

- Tell your family and doctors about your plans to donate. Your next of kin makes the final decision about donation, so make certain family members know of your wish to donate your temporal bones. Please be sure they understand that their cooperation is needed at the time of your death.

- Please keep the Registry informed of any change of address or change in your next of kin.

- Provide up-to-date medical records: The scientific value of your temporal bone donation is greatly enhanced if up-to-date medical records accompany it. Therefore, donors are encouraged to send records of all hearing tests, balance tests, and ear surgery to the Registry. Results of hearing tests (audiograms) that you may have had are extremely valuable. Researchers need your medical records so that they can correlate and link your symptoms to the changes they observe in your donated temporal bones.

Chapter 37

Who's Who in Otologic Health Care

Because of your Meniere's disease, you may visit many health professionals with varied titles, duties, and functions. It might help you to know the following things about them:

Who are these people?

What do they do?

What should you expect from them?

What do their titles mean?

How much education and training have they had?

Few health care professionals receive in-depth education about Meniere's disease or the vestibular system in general. As a consequence, you will meet a large number who may not understand all of your symptoms. The following two quotes illustrate the problems people encounter when seeking treatment:

> "When I told the optometrist about my problems, he just gave me a strange look. Not knowing about Meniere's himself, he did not have any comments."
>
> —D.D., letter to the author, 1997

> "I recently started seeing a psychologist because I am having a hard time dealing with this disease that has so changed my life. And I was quite surprised yesterday to find out how little even he knew about Meniere's. He even asked me if I was sure about the diagnosis because he doesn't understand why my vision problem would be connected to my ear."
>
> —V.T., letter to the author, 1997

Doctors

General Expectations

Generally, you can expect a doctor and his or her office staff to:
• treat you with dignity and courtesy.
• include you in all aspects of your care.
• record your medical history and your current situation.
• examine you.
• select pertinent tests and interpret their results.
• diagnose your problem.
• give you information about the diagnosis and what you need to do.
• discuss all treatment options available.
• refer to another appropriate specialist or clinic if unable to diagnose or treat your problem.
• explain all testing and treatment ahead of time.
• keep accurate written documentation of your condition.
• schedule a follow-up appointment after treatment is started to assess its impact.
• maintain confidentiality of all medical information (except when you have signed the release most health insurance companies insist upon).

Medical Education

The education of medical students in the U.S. differs somewhat from school to school, but in general these students spend their first two years in classrooms studying science and learning some of the skills needed to examine and treat people. Anatomy and physiology, including perhaps one lecture about the ear, are covered during this time.

The second two years are spent among patients in hospitals, clinics, and doctors' offices. During this two-year period, every student gains experience in some areas of medicine but not in others unless he or she specifically chooses to study it. Otolaryngology—head and neck surgery is one of the areas of study not required by all medical schools. Those that do require it may schedule as little as one week of study for otolaryngology.

The average medical student receives an extremely limited introduction to the inner ear. Because of this, you may meet practicing physicians who have almost no knowledge of Meniere's disease or the working of the vestibular system.

M.D. Licensing

In the U.S., all doctors must be licensed to practice medicine by the state they work in. The license verifies that a physician has graduated from an accredited school of medicine and has passed a standardized test showing at least minimum competence. It does not indicate that the doctor has undergone specialty training. The medical license is regulated by the Board of Medicine (or an agency with a similar title) in each state.

Neither M.D. licensing nor advanced certification guarantee in-depth knowledge of the inner ear, particularly vestibular function.

Choosing a Doctor

Your choice of a doctor depends upon your needs. You must decide what you think makes a "good" doctor. Is it someone who is efficient and business-like, one who spends a great deal of time with you, a doctor fresh from residency training with new ideas and methods, an older doctor who has a lot of experience, a doctor who says "don't worry about it," or someone who tells you everything? Do you care only about technical expertise, or is "bedside manner" also important? Decide what attributes you prize most highly before you begin to look.

The best place to start, if you will be doing the selection, is your family doctor. Ask for his or her recommendation. If your doctor makes a recommendation, find out if your doctor or a member of his or her family has been treated by this other doctor. Knowing the basis for your doctor's recommendation could be useful.

Ask friends, relatives, and neighbors if they know of a doctor. If you know any health care professionals socially, ask for their thoughts on the matter. You can get state-by-state flyers from the Vestibular Disorders Association (VEDA) that list doctors interested in vestibular disorders. If you are a VEDA member, you can also ask other members for advice via the VEDA pen pal lists, called Link Lists. Also, look for the Dizzinews and Meniere's mailing lists on the Internet. (See Chapter 39, "Where to Get More Information" for mailing list instructions.)

Try your local library, and look for books like *The Best Doctors in America*, a book that names doctors praised by other doctors. (One drawback may be that the doctors in this book have been chosen by other doctors rather than by the people they have treated.) You should find other helpful books near this one on the library shelf. Also, your librarian may be able to help you get information from the Internet if you don't have a computer.

If you're concerned about the number of lawsuits involving a prospective doctor, you may be able to review complaints and other problems through the agency that regulates medical practice in your state. The State of Florida, for example, has such information available on the Internet. Also, a book called *Questionable Doctors* lists doctors that its authors feel may **not** practice safely.

Note on malpractice: If a health care professional has settled a malpractice claim out of court, it does not automatically mean the professional did anything wrong. For example, settlement may occur because the doctor's insurance company does not want to pay for a jury trial. Most malpractice insurance policies have a clause forcing the insured to settle out of court at the whim of the insurance company. If the insured does not comply, he or she loses insurance coverage.

When someone is found responsible in a malpractice case, keep in mind that the jury did not need to be unanimous in its verdict and that it did not have to be convinced beyond a reasonable doubt; it only had to be sure by a preponderance of the evidence (51 percent sure). A lot of room is left for error.

If you want to be in position to use a certain hospital if the need arises, you must go to a doctor with "privileges" at that hospital. You can get information about privileges by calling a doctor's office and asking. Also, some hospitals have ask-a-nurse and other call-in programs that give the names of their physicians.

If you belong to an HMO or other managed care insurance organization, you will be sent to someone under contract to the organization. The contract is not necessarily made with the best doctor; sometimes it is made with the doctor who accepts the least amount of money from the HMO. This, in and of itself, does not mean the doctor under contract is in any way inferior. Remember that you can go to anyone you want if you are able and willing to pay for it yourself.

Going to Doctors

Most people with hearing loss, tinnitus, and episodes of vertigo start out with their family doctor or visit the emergency room of their local hospital. From there they may be advised to see an otolaryngologist, ENT doctor, otologist, neurotologist, or a neurologist.

Otolaryngologist—Head and Neck Surgeon

An otolaryngologist—head and neck surgeon is a medical doctor who specializes in disorders of the head and neck, especially those related to the ear, nose, and throat. This doctor may also be referred to as an otolaryngologist, otorhinolaryngologist, ear-nose-throat (ENT) doctor, or ENT specialist.

Otolaryngologists don't just specialize in problems of the ear; they do a large assortment of things such as surgery for cancer of the mouth, tongue, throat, or voice box, and plastic surgery for problems such as cleft lips or palates. They treat nose bleeds, nose fractures, and middle ear infections. They remove tonsils and adenoids, perform sinus surgery, and might do allergy work.

Their academic education includes four years of college and four years of medical school. However, these first eight years of higher education might include only extremely limited exposure to inner ear anatomy/physiology and diseases.

Post-medical school training, also called "residency training," in this specialty has a large surgical focus and lasts for at least five years; only a small portion of this is dedicated specifically to otology. After their training is successfully completed, they are eligible to take a certification test known as a "board" given by the American Academy of Otolaryngology. Once they pass the examination, they can refer to themselves as "board certified" and use the title of Fellow of the American College of Surgeons (F.A.C.S.). (Fellow, in this context, means "member.")

If a doctor is "board eligible," it means he or she has completed the required years of residency training but has not taken the certification examination or has not passed it.

In depth (board certification test): The purpose of this test is to provide assurance to the public that a physician specialist certified by a member board of the American Board of Medical Specialties (ABMS) has successfully completed an approved educational program and an evaluation process which includes an examination designed to assess the knowledge, skills, and experience required to provide high-quality patient care in that specialty.

You may encounter another set of terms used to describe a kind of otolaryngologist-in-training, the "otology fellow." A "fellow" traditionally refers to a graduate student to whom an allowance is granted for special study. An otology fellow is an M.D. who has completed a residency in otolaryngology and is studying otology for a year or two while earning a salary.

Otologist

The title of otologist is not given by any agency or organization, and there is no certification examination. In theory, any M.D. could describe himself or herself as an otologist, but in practice the term is generally used by board-certified otolaryngologist—head and neck surgeons who limit their practice to problems and diseases of the **entire** ear. They may or may not have done an additional year or more of training specifically in problems of the ear after their otolaryngology residency was completed.

Neurotologist

Like "otologist," this title is not regulated or granted by any agency or organization. It generally is used by an M.D. who limits practice to problems of the **inner** ear, such as hearing loss, tinnitus, vertigo, and other vestibular or related symptoms. Otolaryngologist—head and neck surgeons may use this title as well as some neurologists who specialize in balance, dizziness, and vertigo problems.

Note: A study done in 1997 questioned members of the American Neurotology Society about the fraction of their practice dedicated to neurotology. Questionnaires were completed by 69.4 percent of the 402 members in the U.S. and Canada. Eighty eight and a half percent called themselves a "vestibular regional authority," but 48 percent spent less than 30 percent of their time with people having a vestibular problem. Only 8 percent spent 81 to 100 percent of their time on vestibular medicine. If this ratio held true for the remainder of the membership who did not respond to the survey, it would mean that as few as 32 neurotologists in the U.S. and Canada devote their practice nearly exclusively to neurotology.

Neurologist

A neurologist is a medical doctor who has undergone four years of residency training in medical problems of the brain, nervous system, and nerves. Neurologists' treatments don't include surgery.

A neurologist may become your primary physician for Meniere's disease or may be used only to help rule out neurological causes of your problem. Many neurological problems can cause dizziness, lightheadedness, and vertigo.

Neurologists that specialize in conditions related to Meniere's disease may call themselves neurotologists, otoneurologists, or otolaryngic neurologists.

Other Specialists

After being seen by an ear specialist, you will most likely be asked to visit and be tested by one or more other specialists such as an allergist, optometrist, ophthalmologist, or neuro-ophthalmologist. The tests can include X-rays and/or an MRI.

Radiologist

A radiologist is a doctor specializing in the reading of X-rays and other body imaging such as CT or CAT scans and MRIs. If you must have X-rays, you will most likely not meet or see the radiologist, but you will receive a bill for his or her services. A technician will actually do the test.

Optometrist

An optometrist is not an M.D. but has completed four years of undergraduate college and is also a graduate of a college of optometry. Optometrists can examine eyes and prescribe glasses and medicines. They don't usually have any training or knowledge about Meniere's disease or any other vestibular disorder.

Ophthalmologist

An ophthalmologist is an M.D. specializing in diseases and surgery of the eyes. Ophthalmologists don't usually have much knowledge of Meniere's disease or any other vestibular problem.

Neuro-Ophthalmologist

A neuro-ophthalmologist is an M.D. who specializes in neurological vision changes. He or she may have some knowledge of Meniere's disease and other vestibular problems

Neurosurgeon

A neurosurgeon is an M.D. who has undergone lengthy residency training learning to surgically treat problems of the brain, nervous system, and nerves. This specialist becomes involved in your care only if vestibular nerve section surgery is to be done.

Anesthesiologist

If you have certain kinds of surgery such as a vestibular nerve section, you will meet an anesthesiologist who will put you to sleep during surgery. An anesthesiologist is a medical doctor who has gone through residency training in the techniques of anesthesia including techniques for general anesthesia, spinal anesthesia, and regional anesthesia. An anesthesiologist also has training in techniques of pain control.

Also in the Doctor's Office

Registered Nurse

A registered nurse (RN) has completed the nursing program at a state-accredited junior college or university, passed a nationally-administered examination, and is licensed to practice nursing by a state board of nursing.

Registered nurses can be considered generalists who know a little bit about many different aspects of health care. They can record your history, assess your current condition, administer medication, take blood, start an IV, change bandages, remove stitches, and teach/inform you about your testing and diagnosis and about treatments such as diet, drugs, and stress reduction.

RNs generally have limited knowledge of the inner ear and its functions unless they have had extra training and education in this area.

Others

Not everyone working at the doctor's office is a nurse. Doctors may use trained employees, medical assistants, licensed practical nurses (LPNs), or registered nurses to complete medical office tasks independently or in a doctor's presence.

Associated Professionals

Audiologist

According to the American Speech-Language-Hearing Association (ASHA), audiologists are hearing health care professionals who specialize in prevention, identification, and assessment of hearing disorders and provide treatment and rehabilitative services.

An audiologist with full credentials can only begin to practice once he or she has completed five to six years of college with a bachelor's and master's degree (or a Ph.D.) in audiology, has spent nine months in supervised practice, and has passed a nationally administered examination. At that point audiologists can use the title Certificate of Clinical Competence in Audiology, abbreviated CCC-A. Most states require licensing and fulfillment of requirements similar to those for the CCC-A for someone to practice audiology.

Audiologists' education and training prepares them to test hearing, administer many different vestibular tests, dispense hearing aids and provide other hearing services and treatments. If you have questions about hearing tests, hearing aids, and other hearing treatments, the audiologist in your doctor's office may be able to answer them.

Physical Therapist

Some symptoms associated with Meniere's disease may make it hard or impossible for you to perform routine tasks. People having any medical or surgical procedure that results in complete loss of vestibular function in one or both ears may have significant symptoms that interfere with their daily routines. Individuals in these situations may be sent to a physical therapist (PT or RPT) and/or an occupational therapist (OT or OTR) for evaluation and treatment.

According to the American Physical Therapy Association, a physical therapist is able to evaluate your joint motion, muscle strength and endurance, functional ability, muscle tone and reflexes, appearance and stability of walking, integrity of sensation and perception, and your performance of daily living activities and developmental activities. Physical therapy techniques include therapeutic exercise, joint mobilization and range-of-motion exercises, relaxation exercises, therapeutic massage, biofeedback, training in the activities of daily living, and ambulation (walking) training.

These therapists enter their profession after completing at least a four-year college course, and many start with a master's degree. They must take and pass a national exam and meet any other requirements of the state board regulating the practice of physical therapists in their state before they can use the title of Registered Physical Therapist (RPT).

Therapists who have had additional training and experience can assess balance, abnormal eye movements, and reactions to position change, and can teach you exercises (vestibular rehabilitation) to accustom your brain to new vestibular signals. However, vestibular rehabilitation is still somewhat new in the U.S.; many of the therapists educated prior to the 1990s will not have studied exercises for vestibular disorders unless they took continuing education courses after graduation. The majority of physical therapists probably know little or nothing about vestibular rehabilitation. Insurance requirements, economic concerns, or other factors may result in your being sent to a therapist with limited vestibular knowledge or experience. If you are sent to a physical therapist, you can ask how long she or he has worked with people with vestibular problems, how many such people he or she has worked with, and if she or he has worked before with anyone in a situation like yours.

Occupational Therapist

According to the Occupational Therapy Association, occupational therapists help people restore and sustain a productive life after setbacks from illness or injury. They also help people cope with developmental disabilities or with changes related to aging.

These therapists use "occupation," meaning "purposeful activity," as a means of preventing, reducing, or overcoming physical, social, and emotional disabilities in people of all ages.

To become an occupational therapist, one must have a bachelor's or master's degree in occupational therapy. To practice in most jobs and most states, occupational therapists must pass a nationally administered test and be licensed. After that, they can use the title of occupational therapist, registered (OTR).

Not all occupational therapists have had education, training, or experience in vestibular disorders. If you are sent for an occupational therapy assessment, you can ask how long she has worked with people with vestibular problems, how many people he has worked with, and if she or he has worked before with anyone in a situation like yours.

Nurse Anesthetist; Certified Registered Nurse Anesthetist (CRNA)

Sometimes anesthesia is given by a nurse anesthetist. He or she is a registered nurse who has gone through two years of training after nursing school and after working as a registered nurse. Also, a nurse anesthetist has passed a national, standardized examination of knowledge about anesthesia.

Note on licensing and/or certification testing: Holding a state license in medicine, nursing, physical therapy, audiology, occupational therapy, or anything else does not guarantee quality. However, dealing only with health care workers who are licensed is one way for you to know that they have met minimum requirements such as schooling and passing a test. If a state board determines that someone should stop practicing in a health care profession, he or she will not be able to get work in that profession anywhere in the U.S. When unlicensed people, some with scant education and training, replace licensed health care professionals, this safeguard is lost.

Mental Health Professionals

Some people with Meniere's disease feel an acute loss of control and, possibly, depression. Seeing a psychiatrist or psychologist may be recommended.

Psychiatrist

A psychiatrist is an M.D. who specializes in psychiatry after completing a psychiatric residency training program. A psychiatrist usually does not have any specific training in Meniere's disease or other vestibular disorders.

Psychologist

A psychologist is someone with college degrees in psychology. He or she will usually have a Ph.D. in some area of psychology and will have spent eight or more years studying psychology in college. It would be unusual if this professional had any training or experience in Meniere's disease or any other vestibular disorder.

Summary

While dealing with Meniere's disease, you may encounter many health care professionals. Don't assume they know anything about Meniere's disease or the vestibular system. Ask if they have been trained in this area and if they are seeing other patients with symptoms and problems like yours.

References

_____. *The American College Encyclopedic Dictionary, Vol. 1.* Chicago: Spencer Press, 1957.

_____. *The Official ABMS Directory of Board Certified Medical Specialists, Vol. 3: Otolaryngologists.* 28th edition. Illinois: Marquis, 1995.

American Neurotology Society, "The American Neurotology Society," http://itsa.ucsf.edu/~ajo/ANS/Policies/Policy.html. June 6, 1997.

American Occupational Therapy Association (AOTA), "Member Information," http://www.aota.org/membinfo.html. June 6, 1997.

American Academy of Otolaryngology—Head and Neck Surgery. "What Is an Otolaryngologist—Head and Neck Surgeon?" (public service brochure), 1994.

American Speech-Language-Hearing Association (ASHA), *Membership and Certification Handbook—Audiology,* 1994.

Cohen, H., Rubin, A.M., and Gombash, L. "The Team Approach to Treatment of the Dizzy Patient." *Archives of Physical Medicine and Rehabilitation,* 73:703-708, 1992.

Naifeh, S., and Smith, G.W. *The Best Doctors in America*. South Carolina: Woodward/White, 1994.

Wolfe, S., Gabay, M., McCarthy, P., Bame, A., and Adler, B.M. *Questionable Doctors: A Public Citizen Health Research Group Report*, March 1996.

Chapter 38

Insurance

If you have Meniere's disease, you will find it useful to know something about health insurance coverage offered by traditional insurers, Health Maintenance Organizations (HMOs), Preferred Provider Organizations (PPOs), the Consolidated Omnibus Budget Reconciliation Act of 1985 (COBRA), Medicare, and Medicaid. You may also want to know about disability insurance, including Social Security Disability Insurance.

Health Insurance

Health insurance comes in many varieties and with a staggering number of rules and regulations. It can be divided generally into traditional insurance coverage, PPOs, HMOs, Medicaid, and Medicare. The information below will give you an overview of health insurance. Refer to your insurance policy for any specific information you may need about benefits, rules, and regulations.

Traditional Health Insurance

With traditional health insurance, you pay a monthly premium, and the insurance company pays a percentage of your medical bills. The percentage the insurance company pays is determined by the individual policy. Usually, you are responsible for the first $250 to $500 of charges (the deductible) each year. After the deductible limit is reached, the insurer will usually pay 80 percent of a "reasonable and customary" charge, and you will pay 20 percent. With this kind of policy, the insurer places no restrictions on which doctor you see. Generally, this type of health insurance is the most expensive.

PPO Health Insurance

Preferred provider organization (PPO) health insurance usually allows you to visit any doctor in any place, but your out-of-pocket expense will be lower if you choose someone on the PPO's list of preferred providers. The list generally includes doctors, hospitals, labs, radiology offices, and other health-care professionals and agencies.

A typical arrangement is for the PPO to pay 90 percent and for you to pay 10 percent of the bills for treatment by a preferred provider. If you choose a non-preferred provider for treatment, the PPO will pay less, and you will pay more.

HMO Health Insurance

Insurance from a health maintenance organization (HMO) involves a membership contract between you and the organization. By joining, you are allowing the HMO to decide what health care you will receive and from whom. If you want the HMO to pay for your medical bills, your choice is limited to those providers, facilities, and hospitals under contract with that particular HMO. Your bills will not be paid if you seek care outside of the HMO while you are living at home. Different rules apply when you are traveling away from home.

Some HMOs hire their own doctors and specialists and buy or create their own clinics and hospitals. Other HMOs may hire MDs and make contracts with hospitals and other health-care agencies that are independent of the HMO.

Most HMOs have stringent rules about using emergency room services. They do not want to pay emergency room rates for non-emergency problems. For example, here is one insurance company's list of health conditions or situations that constitute an emergency:

• uncontrolled bleeding
• severe burns
• seizure or loss of consciousness
• broken bones
• severe shortness of breath
• inability to swallow
• suspected drug overdose or poisoning
• chest pain or severe squeezing sensation in the chest
• stroke symptoms such as sudden paralysis, suddenly slurred speech, numbness or paralysis of arm or leg, lack of responsiveness, severe headache

If you have Meniere's disease and belong to an HMO, you should ask your doctor ahead of time if and when you should go to the emergency room for a Meniere's attack. Sometimes HMOs have refused to pay emergency room bills for problems they did not define as emergencies.

Medicare

Medicare is a kind of U.S. Federal health insurance available to people receiving Social Security retirement benefits or Social Security disability benefits.

People are automatically eligible for Medicare after receiving Social Security disability benefits for two years. Enrollment in Medicare decreases the monthly disability check by the relatively small cost of the Medicare premium.

Medicare coverage includes various options, including using an HMO. Get and read current Medicare publications before making any decisions about health insurance coverage. Keep in mind that if you don't enroll for Medicare when it is first offered to you, you will pay a much higher premium if you enroll later.

Medicaid

Medicaid is a kind of governmental health insurance for the indigent. This insurance is funded by both the U.S. Federal government and individual state governments. Because of this setup, Medicaid eligibility and benefits can differ significantly from state to state.

Generally, to qualify for Medicaid your monthly income must be very low and your bank accounts must be very small.

Some Common Health Insurance Terms

Authorization, pre-authorization, or *referral* are terms used by insurers to mean the process of granting official permission to see a specialist or have a test or procedure done that can't be done by your primary care doctor. This permission may be given verbally or in writing. Different health plans have different rules; ask about them when you are told to go for specialty care or testing.

Pre-certification is another term used to mean the process of getting official permission from your insurance company for something such as an MRI (or other equally expensive test) or surgery. Pre-certification has become routine with most insurers, including Medicare, Medicaid, PPOs, and traditional health insurers.

A *co-payment* or *co-insurance* refers to a fixed amount of money you pay for a visit to the doctor's office, usually $5 to $10, in addition to the money paid for the visit by your insurance.

A *deductible* is the total amount of money you must spend on your annual health care bills before your insurance company begins to pay. Only health care covered by your insurance policy counts toward the total.

In-patient and *out-patient* are important terms because some insurance companies pay at one rate for out-patient tests and procedures and at another rate for in-patient. These two terms have blurred significantly over the last several years. Staying overnight in the hospital used to define the difference; now you may be considered an out-patient even if your hospital stay is as much as 23 hours and includes one night.

Medically necessary is a term used to describe whether or not your insurance company considers a test, office visit, procedure, or treatment necessary given your diagnosis and condition. Whether or not your primary doctor or specialist thinks it is needed is not the question.

Usual and customary, usual and prevailing, or *allowable* are terms used to refer to the amount of money the insurance company says something should cost. This is not necessarily what your doctor charges or what anyone else has charged you.

Privacy Issue

Insurance companies almost always insist upon having full access to your medical records as a pre-requisite to paying your claim. In many cases, you will be asked to sign a form giving your doctor permission to send any requested part of your medical record to your insurance company. The only way this situation can be avoided is for you to pay for your own care.

Problem Areas

Generally speaking, most people don't have health insurance problems specifically related to Meniere's disease. There are, however, two exceptions: computerized dynamic posturography (CDP) and facial nerve monitoring during vestibular nerve section surgery.

In 1997, the cost of CDP generally fell in the $400 to $600 range and was considered by some insurance companies as unnecessary or unproven/experimental and not something these companies wanted to pay for. (In the author's personal experience, insurance companies seldom raise these objections when a test or treatment is inexpensive.)

Facial nerve monitoring is a tool surgeons use to help prevent injury to the facial nerve during some inner ear surgeries. Some insurance companies pay at a very low rate for this service, particularly when compared to other parts of the hospital bill.

People in your doctor's office may be able to provide information about these two areas.

Health Insurance if You Leave Your Job

If you are unable to perform your job and leave work of your own accord or are fired, you may be eligible to maintain your employee health insurance policy through the Consolidated Omnibus Budget Reconciliation Act of 1985 (COBRA).This Federal law requires any employer with 20 or more employees to offer the continuation of health insurance after an employee has left a job. The coverage must usually be provided for 18 months, possibly more under certain circumstances. This act does not require the employer to pay for the coverage, only to provide the departing employee with the opportunity to buy it. In order to qualify, you must sign up within 60 days of leaving your job.

Disability Insurance

Only a small number of people with a diagnosis of Meniere's disease will become disabled to the point of being unable to continue working for pay. According to the 1995 annual report of the National Institute on Deafness and Other Communication Disorders, during 1994 only an estimated 7,600 people throughout the U.S. received Social Security benefits (Social Security Disability Insurance payments and Supplemental Security Income payments combined) for balance problems, including those caused by Meniere's disease. A larger number received benefits for disability caused by hearing problems.

Note about working: Try to continue working as long as you safely can. Usually, Social Security disability payments and private disability insurance will not come close to matching your normal paycheck. Also, even if you qualify for Social Security disability, you will not be eligible for health insurance from Medicare until two years later.

Disability benefits may be available from a private insurance policy and/or the government via the Social Security Administration for people unable to keep their jobs.

Benefits from a private insurance policy differ from situation to situation. Most policies have a choice of elimination periods (the varying periods of time that must go by before certain benefits begin) and different amounts of payment. These policies are usually set up to cover you for a short time until you qualify for Social Security disability benefits.

If you did not buy a private disability insurance policy on your own, check to see if you have such coverage through your employer. (Sometimes such coverage is referred to as "short term disability.")

Social Security

Note: This section of the book contains quotes, not the entire texts, from Social Security publications. You should obtain and read current Social Security publications in their entirety before applying for or making decisions about Social Security. See "For More Information" later in this chapter for Social Security's central phone numbers and its World Wide Web address, or visit your local branch.

Disability Definition

According to the Social Security Administration,

"Disability under Social Security is based on your inability to work. You will be considered disabled if you are unable to do any kind of work for which you are suited and your disability is expected to last for at least a year or to result in death."

Different Social Security Programs

The Social Security Administration oversees two different programs related to disability, Social Security Disability Insurance (SSDI) and Supplemental Security Income (SSI). A person's disability is determined by the same process for each program, but the financial eligibility differs. Financial eligibility for Social Security disability is based on how much you have contributed to Social Security over time, and SSI disability payments are made on the basis of your current financial need. (Your contributions to Social Security are not taken into account.) Social Security Publication No. 05-11000 has more information.

These two Social Security programs are set up to begin six months after the start of the kind of disability defined above. It is assumed that people will have their own contingency plans to support them during a disability of less than one year.

Although the disability must go on for at least a year to qualify, your benefits could begin to accumulate prior to the one-year date. For example, suppose that in January 1998 you became unable to work. In June 1998, you applied for Social Security benefits. A year later, in June 1999, benefits are approved. In this case, you will be paid retroactively (in a lump sum) for each month between June 1998 and June 1999, and you will also begin to receive ongoing monthly benefits. If your initial application were rejected, *and* you chose to appeal, *and* you used a lawyer during the appeal stage, *and* you won your appeal, a predetermined percentage of this lump sum would go for the lawyer's services.

When Do You Apply?

There is no general answer to the question of when to apply for

Social Security disability benefits. A diagnosis of Meniere's disease does not automatically make you eligible for a disability benefit; you must also meet the Social Security Administration's definition of "disabled." Someone who fits the definition and has been unable to work for five months or more would have the greatest chance of obtaining disability benefits.

How to Apply

You can apply at a Social Security office by phone or mail. According to a Social Security publication, "Social Security disability benefits will not begin until the sixth full month of disability. This waiting period begins with the first full month after the date we decide your disability began." The application process will usually require 60 to 90 days.

What You Need for the Application

For the application process, you need all of the following:

- names, addresses, and phone numbers of doctors, hospitals, clinics, and institutions that treated you; dates of treatment
- names of all the medications you are taking
- medical records from your doctors, therapists, hospitals, clinics, and caseworkers, including laboratory and test results
- a summary of where you worked in the past 15 years and the kind of work you did
- a copy of your W-2 Form (Wage and Tax Statement), or if you are self-employed, your Federal tax return for the past year

Who Decides if You Are Disabled?

According to a Social Security publication called "Social Security Disability Benefits," the Social Security office will review your application:

> "to see if you are eligible to apply for disability benefits. These include such factors as whether you have worked long enough and recently enough to qualify for disability benefits, your age, and, if you are applying for benefits as a family member, your relationship to the worker. The office will then send your application to the Disability Determination Services (DDS) office in your state. There, a decision will be made as to whether you are disabled under the Social Security law.

> "In the DDS office, a team consisting of a physician (or psychologist) and a disability evaluation specialist will consider

all the facts in your case and decide if you are disabled. They will use the medical evidence from your doctors and from hospitals, clinics, or institutions where you have been treated.

"On the medical report forms, your doctors or other sources are asked for a medical history of your condition: what is wrong with you; when it began; how it limits your activities; what the medical tests have shown; and what treatment has been provided. They are also asked for information about your ability to do work-related activities, such as walking, sitting, lifting, and carrying. They are not asked to decide whether you are disabled.

"Additional medical information may be needed before the DDS team can decide your case. If it is not available from your current medical sources, you may be asked to take a special examination called a consultative examination. Your doctor or the medical facility where you have been treated is the preferred source to perform this examination. Social Security will pay for the examination or any other additional medical tests you may need, and for certain travel expenses related to it."

SSA officials use a Social Security publication entitled, "Disability Evaluation Under Social Security" to help determine disability. One passage of this document pertains specifically to Meniere's disease, as follows:

"Meniere's disease is characterized by paroxysmal attacks of vertigo, tinnitus, and fluctuating hearing loss. Remissions are unpredictable and irregular, but may be long-lasting; hence, the severity of impairment is best determined after prolonged observation and serial re-examinations. The diagnosis of a vestibular disorder requires a comprehensive neuro-otolaryngologic examination with a detailed description of the vertiginous episodes, including notation of frequency, severity, and duration of the attacks. Pure tone and speech audiometry, with the appropriate special examinations, such as Bekesy audiometry, are necessary. (Bekesy audiometry allows the person being tested to control the intensity of the testing tones by pushing a button.) Vestibular function is assessed by positional and caloric testing, preferably by electronystagmography."

If Your Claim Is Denied

According to another SSA publication, "The Appeals Process,"

"If your claim is denied or you disagree with any other decision we make, you may appeal the decision. The Social Security office will help you complete the paperwork.

"There are four levels of appeal. If you disagree with the decision at one level, you may appeal to the next level. You have 60 days from the time you receive the decision to file an appeal to the next level. We assume that you receive the decision five days after the date on it, unless you can show us that you received it later. For more information about appeals, ask for the fact sheet, (Publication No. 05-10041)."

Should I Hire a Lawyer?

This is a choice you must make for yourself, but keep in mind that you can't use a lawyer unless you have been turned down by Social Security and have decided to request an appeal. If you use a lawyer, you will be asked to give him or her a percentage of the money you may be owed by the Social Security Administration.

For More Information

According to Social Security,

"You can get more information 24 hours a day by calling Social Security's toll-free number: 1-800-772-1213. You can speak to a service representative between the hours of 7 a.m. and 7 p.m. on business days. Pre-recorded information and services also are available during and after normal business hours.

"If you want to speak to a representative, it's best to call later in the week and later in the month. When you call, have your Social Security number handy.

"Hearing-impaired callers using TTY equipment can reach Social Security between 7 a.m. and 7 p.m. weekdays by calling 1-800-325-0778."

Here are some booklets you can obtain from the Social Security Administration:

• "SSI" (Publication No. 05-11000)—explains the Supplemental Security Income program, which provides a basic income to people who are 65 or older, disabled, or blind, and have limited income and resources
• "Benefits for Children with Disabilities" (Publication No. 05-10026)—explains benefits available to children with disabilities

- "Working While Disabled . . . How We Can Help" (Publication No. 05-10095)—explains work incentives for Social Security and SSI beneficiaries

    Social Security information is also available to users of the Internet. To view Social Security information on the World Wide Web of the Internet, go to http://www.ssa.gov.

Meniere's Disease and Social Security

Someone diagnosed with Meniere's disease faces the following difficulties when trying to qualify for Social Security disability benefits:

- First and foremost is the unpredictable nature of the disease. Nobody, including your doctor, will be able to predict what your future holds.

- The Social Security Administration's definition of Meniere's disease includes hearing loss, something not present in everyone with the diagnosis. (Some doctors may diagnose Meniere's disease whether or not you have a hearing loss.)

- Sometimes the medical record kept by your doctor does not indicate all the problems you are having. This medical record is read by Social Security officials to help them decide your status. People with Meniere's disease already know how they feel, what in their lives has changed, and what their abilities are. Physicians, on the other hand, don't really know how it "feels;" they usually can't see how a patient's life has been affected and, most importantly, can't measure disability objectively, such as with a test.

What You Can Do to Avoid Problems

You can do the following things to avoid problem with your application:

- Tell your doctor what is happening to you. You are the only one who knows how you feel and how your functioning has been affected. This must be communicated to your doctor. Keep a journal of your problems, the number of attacks, their violence, if there is vomiting, how long you are unable to function after the attack, how many days you are taking off from work. No test will show your disability; you must report it to your doctor. Do not assume someone knows what you are going through; every case of Meniere's is different.

- Get a true advocate. Sometimes the medical record is a problem because your doctor doesn't believe you or thinks your symptoms are not as bad as you say. If this becomes the case, you need to look for someone more experienced in dealing with inner ear problems who can act as an advocate not a skeptic.

- Seek follow-up care. An on-going medical record is needed to retain Social Security disability benefits. To maintain such a record, you must see a doctor at somewhat regular intervals.

Disability Planning

Statistically, you are not likely to become totally disabled by Meniere's disease. However, to improve your chances of avoiding financial disaster, here are some steps you can take:

- Save enough money to last through six or more months of unemployment.
- Acquire a disability policy that begins nearly immediately since Social Security does not pay immediately even if you qualify for it quickly.
- Try to accumulate sick time, holiday time, and vacation time at work if you have those benefits.
- Attempt to get a few months ahead on your car payments and the like.
- Buy insurance. If you are currently well and don't have some type of private disability insurance to replace your salary, you might want to consider it. Disability insurance can be bought through an insurance agent, at work, or directly from an insurance company, or it may be offered by an organization you belong to such as a credit union or professional organization. Many items you buy, such as cars and houses, may be sold with an option for disability coverage. Insurance coverage for credit card balances may also be available.

Not many people with Meniere's disease become too disabled to work. If you can't work, you can try to collect disability benefits. For those who can afford it, insurance, both health and disability, can mean the difference between sinking economically or staying afloat.

References

_____. Public Health Service, U.S. Department of Health and Human Services, National Institutes of Health, *Research in Human Communication: 1995 Annual Report of the National Institute on Deafness and Other Communication Disorders.* NIDCD:Bethesda, Md., 1997.

_____. Social Security Administration, U.S. Department of Health and Human Services. "Social Security Disability Benefits." SSA Publication No. 05-10029, May 1996.

_____. Social Security Administration, U.S. Department of Health and Human Services. "Disability Evaluation Under Social Security." SSA Publication No. 64-039, Jan. 1995.

Cohen, H., Ewell, L.R., and Jenkins, H. "Disability in Meniere's Disease." *Archives of Otolaryngology—Head and Neck Surgery,* 121:29-33, 1995.

Delk, J.H. *Comprehensive Dictionary of Audiology.* Sioux City Iowa: The Hearing Aid Journal, 1973.

Kinney, S.E. Sandridge, S.A., and Newman, C.W. "Long-Term Effects of Meniere's Disease on Hearing and Quality of Life." *American Journal of Otology,* 18: 67-73, 1997.

Parnes, L.S., and Sindwani, R. "Impact of Vestibular Disorders on Fitness to Drive: A Census of the American Neurotology Society." *American Journal of Otology,* 18:79-85, 1997.

Chapter 39

Where to Get More Information

Your first source of information about Meniere's disease and its diagnosis, treatment, and effects should always be your doctor and members of his or her staff (particularly the audiologist for questions about hearing). Your pharmacist can tell you about drugs and drug interactions. Additional information can also be found through libraries and from patient support organizations, the Internet (whether or not you own a computer), and other people with similar problems.

Libraries

The library has always been a good place to go for information. This is true even in the age of the Internet. You can find information about Meniere's disease at your local public library, hospital library, college library, and the closest medical school library.

Start with the librarian at your local library. She or he can make suggestions to help get you started. If the local library does not have the information you are looking for, the reference librarian or another librarian may be able to get it. Most libraries borrow books they don't own from libraries that have them (interlibrary loan). They can also help with access to the Internet.

Hospitals sometimes maintain medical libraries for their doctors and staffs, and sometimes these libraries are available for public use. On occasion, a hospital will have a library or a library section devoted to public education. These hospital libraries usually have a modest selection of books and scientific journals. Be prepared to do your own looking since hospital librarians may not have much time to assist you; their primary mission is to serve the hospital staff.

The local junior college may also have useful books and journals, particularly if it has a health care program for registered nurses, respiratory therapists, physical therapy assistants, or other health professionals. Many four-year colleges and universities also have books, magazines, and scientific journals related to health care.

Medical schools usually have well-stocked medical libraries, and borrowing privileges may be available to the public. The information at these libraries will most likely be meant for graduate physicians, medical students, and students of other professional schools (nursing, audiology, physical therapy, pharmacy, occupational therapy, dentistry) associated with the college. If you are interested in reading medical and other health care journals, go prepared to make copies; journals usually can't be checked out of the library but must be used on the premises. Although medical school librarians may not have time to help you as much as public librarians, most of the medical libraries include displays and brochures explaining where things are and how to find them.

Some private clinics also make vestibular materials available to the public. For example, if you live near Los Angeles, you might find what you are looking for in the otology library at the House Ear Institute.

Organizations

Many organizations offer information to people about Meniere's disease. Professional organizations, patient support organizations, research organizations, and the Federal government all distribute such information.

The Vestibular Disorders Association (VEDA) and the National Institute on Deafness and Other Communication Disorders (NIDCD) Information Clearinghouse are two good places to start. VEDA has a large collection of non-technical printed information as well audiotapes and videotapes. It sends and receives e-mail and has a substantial Internet web site.

Patient support organizations exist nationally and locally. National and international groups such as VEDA, Self-Help for the Hard of Hearing People, Inc. (SHHH), and the Acoustic Neuroma Association have general information as well as information about local support groups.

In the list below, lines containing the @ symbol are e-mail addresses. Lines beginning with http:// are addresses of sites on the World Wide Web of the Internet.

Patient Support Organizations

Acoustic Neuroma Association
P.O. Box 12402; Atlanta, GA 30355
Phone: (404) 237-8023; Fax (404) 237-2704
anausa@aol.com; http://www.anausa.org

Acoustic Neuroma Association of Canada
P.O. Box 369; Edmonton, AB T5J 2J6
Voice/TTY (403) 428-3383 or 3384; Toll-Free (800) 561-2622
(Canada only)
anac@compusmart.ab.ca

Acoustic Neuroma Association of Australasia
PO Box 21; Georges Hall, NSW 2198; Australia
(02) 9708 2695

American Autoimmune Related Diseases Association
Michigan National Bank Building; 15475 Gratiot Ave.
Detroit, MI 48205
Phone: (313) 371-8600; Toll-Free: (800) 598-4668
Fax: (313) 371-6002
aarda@aol.com

American Tinnitus Association
P.O. Box 5; Portland, OR 97207
(503) 248-9985; Fax: (503) 248-0024
tinnitus@ata.org; http://www.ata.org

Association of Late-Deafened Adults (ALDA)
10310 Main St. #274; Fairfax, VA 22030
TTY: (404) 289-1596; Fax: (404) 284-6862
http://www.alda.org

Autoimmune Inner Ear Disease Association (AIEDA)
c/o Douglas Lynch; 23713 Ashwood Place; Valencia, CA 91345
dougl@advancedbionics.com

Brain Injury Association
1776 Mass. Ave. NW, #100; Washington, DC 20036
Phone: (202) 296-6443; Toll-Free: (800) 444-6443

Center for Stress-Related Tinnitus and Hyperacusis Disorders
Kenneth Greenspan, M.D.; 348 E. 51st. St.; New York, NY 10022
Phone: (212) 888-5140; Fax: (212) 888-5612

The CFIDS (Chronic Fatigue and Immune Dysfunction Syndrome)
  Association of America
P.O. Box 220398; Charlotte, NC 28222-0398
Toll-Free: (800) 442-3437; Information (900) 988-2343
Fax: (704) 365-9755
cfids@vnet.net; http://cfids.org/cfids

Cochlear Implant Club International
5335 Wisconsin Ave. NW, Suite 440
Washington, D.C. 20015-2003
Voice/TTY: (202) 895-2781 Fax: (202) 895-2782
http://www.cici.org

Commissie Ménière NVVS
Postbus 9505; 3506GM Utrecht; The Netherlands
Phone: 31/4749786

Danmarks Ménièreförening
Abildgärdsparken 20; 3460 Birkerød; Danmark
Phone/Fax: 45-42-815647

Entraide Ménière
Ruelle Marschal, 5; 1450 Chastre; Belgium
Phone: (+32) 10- 65.00.67

Finnish Ménière Society
Eero Aantaa; Tuurintie 3A14; 20100 Turku; Finland
Phone and Fax: (358)- 2-2505115

Hyperacusis Network
Dan Malcore; 444 Edgewood Drive; Green Bay, WI 54302-4873
Phone: (414) 468-4667; Fax: (414) 432-3321
hyacusis@netnet.net
http://www.visi.com/~minuet/hearing/hyperacusis/index.html

International Ménière Federation
Weikantstraat 9; 1800 Vilvoorde; Belgium
Phone/Fax: 32-2-2676676

Kings Valley Collies (service dogs)
39968 Ward Road; Kings Valley, OR 97361
Phone: (541) 929-2100; Fax: (541) 929-4593
kvav@aol.com

Ménièregruppen
Hörselskadades Sist. i Stockholm; Box 20113; 104 60 Stockholm
Sweden
Phone: 46.8.702.3085; Fax: 46.8.642.59.30

Meniere's Australia, Inc.
P.O. Box 202; Moonah, Tasmania 7009
Phone: (03) 62341494; Fax: (03) 62781520
meniere@tassie.net.au; http://www.tassie.net.au/~meniere

Meniere's Network and The Ear Foundation
1817 Patterson St.; Nashville, TN 37203
Voice/TDD: (615) 329-7807 in Tennessee
Voice/TDD: (800) 545-HEAR elsewhere
earfyi@aol.com; http://www.theearfound.com/

Meniere's Society U.K.
98 Maybury Road; Woking; Surrey GU21 5HX
Phone: 01483 740597; Minicom and Fax: 01483 771207

Meniere's Support Group of Victoria
7 St. Kilda St.; Mount Eliza; Victoria 3930; Australia
Phone: (03) 9775-2972
menieres@outeast.cyberspace.net.au

Morbus Ménière Selbsthilfegruppe
Katanienweg 5; 7054 Korb; Germany

National Ataxia Association
15500 Wayzata Blvd. #750; Wayzata, MN 55391
(612) 473-7666; Fax: (612) 473-9289
naf@mr.net; http://www ataxia.org

National Chronic Fatigue Syndrome Association
3521 Broadway, Suite 222; Kansas City, MO 64111
(816) 931-4777; Fax: (816) 524-6782

National Head Injury Foundation
1776 Massachusetts Ave. N.W. #100; Washington, D.C. 20036
(202) 296-6443; (800) 444-6443

National Information Center on Deafness
Gallaudet University
800 Florida Ave. NE; Washington, DC 20002-3695
Voice: (202) 651-5051; TDD: (202) 651-5052
nicd@gallux.gallaudet.edu; http://www.gallaudet.edu:80/~nicd/

National Mental Health Association
1021 Prince Street; Alexandria, VA 22314-2971
(703) 684-7722; Fax: (703) 684-7722
nmhainfo@aol.com; http://www.nmha.org

National Multiple Sclerosis Society
Public Policy Office
1100 New York Ave., NW, Ste. 1015; Washington, DC 20005-3934
(202) 408-1500; Fax: (202) 408-0696
http://www.nmss.org/

National Organization for Rare Disorders (NORD)
PO Box 8923; New Fairfield, CT 06812-8923
(203) 746-6518; (800) 999-6673; Fax: (203) 746-6481
orphan@nord-rdb.com; http://www.rarediseases.org

National Stroke Association
96 Inverness Dr. E., Ste. I; Englewood, CO 80112-5112
Phone: (303) 649-9299; Fax: (303) 649-1328
http://www.stroke.org/

Neuro-Optometric Rehabilitation Association (NORA)
PO Box 1408; Guilford, CT 06437
(203) 453-2222
http://www.noravc.com/

New South Wales Meniere's Support Group
PO Box 1077; Bowral, NSW 2576; Australia
Phone: (04) 861-3751
nswmsg@hinet.net.au

Self-Help for Hard of Hearing People, Inc. (SHHH)
7910 Woodmont Ave.; Bethesda, Maryland 20814
Voice: (301) 657-2248; TDD: (301) 657-2249; Fax: (301) 913-9413
http://www.shhh.org/

SHHH Australia
1334 Pacific Highway; Turramurra, NSW 2074
Voice/TTY: (02) 9144-7586; Fax: (02) 9449-2381

Tinnitus Association of Canada
23 Ellis Park Road; Toronto, ON M6S 2V4
(416) 762-1490

Vestibular Disorders Association (VEDA)
P.O. Box 4467; Portland, OR 97208-4467
(503) 229-7705 (24-hour answering machine)
(800) 837-8428 (24-hour answering machine); Fax: (503) 229-8064
veda@vestibular.org; http://www.vestibular.org

Professional Organizations

American Academy of Neurology (AAN)
2221 University Ave. S.E., Ste. 335; Minneapolis, MN 55414
(800) 879-1960; (612) 623-8115; Fax: (612) 623-2491
aan@aan.com; http://www.aan.com

American Academy of Otolaryngology—Head and Neck Surgery
One Prince Street; Alexandria, VA 22314
Phone (703) 836-4444; TTY: (703) 519-1585; Fax: (703) 683-5100
entnews@aol.com; http://www.entnet.org/

American Occupational Therapy Association
4720 Montgomery Lane; Bethesda, MD 20814-3425
Voice: (301) 652-2682; Fax: (301) 652-7711
http://www.aota.org/

American Physical Therapy Association
1111 N. Fairfax Street; Alexandria, VA 22314
Phone: (703) 684-2782, extension 8555; Toll-Free: (800) 999-2782
TTY: (703) 684-6748; Fax: (703) 684-7343
ablake@apta.org; http://www.apta.org/

American Psychiatric Association
Division of Public Affairs
1400 K Street, NW; Washington, DC 20005
Phone: (202) 682-6000
http://www.psych.org/index.html

American Psychological Association
750 First Street., NE; Washington, DC 20002-4242
Phone: (202) 336-5500; Toll-Free: (800) 374-2721
http://www.apa.org/

American-Speech-Language-Hearing Association (ASHA)
10801 Rockville Pike; Rockville, MD 20852-3279
Toll-Free: (800) 498-2071; Voice: (301) 897-5700
TTY: (301) 897-0157; Fax: (301) 571-0457
http://www.asha.org/

Deafness Research Foundation
15 W. 39th St.; New York, NY 10018
Voice/TDD: (212) 684-6556; Voice/TDD: (800) 535-DEAF
drf1@village.ios.com; http://village.ios.com/~drf1/index.html

National Organization for Hearing Research
225 Haverford Ave. #1; Narberth, PA 19072
Voice/TDD: (610) 664-3135

U. S. Government

Hereditary Hearing Impairment Resource Registry (NIDCD)
555 N. 30th St.; Omaha, NE 68131-9909
Voice/TDD: (800) 320-1171
nidcd-hhirr@boystown.org; http://www.boystown.org/hhirr

National Library of Medicine
8600 Rockville Pike; Bethesda, MD 20894
Voice: (888) 346-3656
publicinfo@nlm.nih.gov; http://www.nlm.nih.gov/

NIDCD Information Clearinghouse
1 Communication Ave.; Bethesda, MD 20892-3456
Voice: (800) 241-1044; TDD/TT: (800) 241-1055; Fax: (301) 907-8830
nidcdinfo@nidcd.nih.gov; http://www.nih.gov/nidcd/

NIDCD National Temporal Bone, Hearing, and Balance Pathology Resource Registry
Massachusetts Eye and Ear Infirmary
243 Charles St.; Boston, MA 02114-3096
Voice: (800) 822-1327; Voice: (617) 573-3711
TDD: (617) 573-3888; Fax: (617) 573-3838
tbregistry@meei.harvard.edu; http://www.tbregistry.org

Social Security Administration
(Check the telephone Yellow Pages for information on your local Social Security branch office.)
Voice: (800) 772-1213; TTY: (800) 325-0778
http://www.ssa.gov/reach.htm

Internet

If you have a computer and Internet access, you are probably already familiar with news groups, electronic mailing lists, web pages, and other electronic communication modes. Most of these modes can provide access to information about Meniere's disease.

If you don't have a computer, try your local library. Most libraries have Internet access, and librarians can help you find things on the Internet.

If you don't have a computer, you can also ask neighbors and relatives who may have Internet access or know someone who does. Most people using the Internet would probably be happy to help you find information; part of their fun is the hunt.

Also, your town may have a "cyber cafe," a retail business offering Internet access in a coffee house setting.

What Can You Find on the Internet?

The Internet includes an enormous amount of information. The U.S. Federal government has huge sites, including those of the Social Security Administration, the National Institute on Deafness and Other Communication Disorders (NIDCD), the National Institutes of Health (NIH), the National Library of Medicine (NLM), the Library of Congress and more. Information from many organizations, colleges and universities, hospitals, doctors, and individuals are available on the Internet. Many publishers of professional medical journals list the tables of contents of their journal issues; some even include summaries of the articles.

Government forms and publications are available "on-line" including booklets from the Social Security Administration. You can download them and print them immediately without writing a letter and waiting for a reply.

Books in print are listed at the Library of Congress Internet site, and medical books in print are listed at the NLM site.

A handful of universities have posted on-line textbooks containing basic anatomy and physiology of the ear and other ear information, including graphics, at their web sites.

If you want to read current scientific papers on Meniere's disease and other topics, you can look for abstracts and bibliographic information on the Internet using MEDLINE, a database of the NLM. On June 26, 1997, the NLM announced free access to MEDLINE via a World Wide Web service called PubMed. MEDLINE contains more than 8.8 million references to articles published in 3,800 biomedical journals. Many of these references include 300-word abstracts as well as the names of titles, authors, publishers, and other bibliographic information. You can search MEDLINE at home or at work using your own computer and Internet connection, or you can use on-line services at libraries or other institutions offering web access to the public. To connect to PubMed or to find out more about it and other NLM services, go to the web page at http://www.nlm.nih.gov. MEDLINE and related databases are used by health care professionals and researchers as well as the general public.

Other People with Meniere's

How do you find other people with Meniere's disease?

- First, ask at your doctor's office. (If your ear specialist doesn't know of anyone else with similar problems, he or she isn't seeing many people with Meniere's or other vestibular problems, and you might want to re-evaluate going to this doctor).

- Ask your friends and relatives if they know of anyone with Meniere's, and you might also try the clergy.

- If you are a VEDA member, you can ask other members for suggestions, stories, and advice via the VEDA pen pal lists, called Link Lists. VEDA's addresses are listed in the "Organizations" section earlier in this chapter.

- If you have Internet access, you can find others with similar problems through an electronic mailing list such as the Meniere's Discussion Group or a news group such as alt.support.tinnitus.

To join an electronic mailing list related to Meniere's disease, you must subscribe (for free) via e-mail. You must follow subscription directions exactly since the entire process is handled by a computer, not a person. Unless you write the appropriate command in the correct place with the correct spelling, your e-mail subscription request will fail. If you are unsuccessful the first time, check your word placement and spelling. Delete all extraneous material, such as your automated signature lines, from your message. Here are examples:

Dizzinews Mailing List
To: majordomo@samurai.com
From: your e-mail address
Subject: (leave blank)
Message: subscribe dizzinews

Meniere's Discussion Group
To: requests@smtp.cochlea.com
From: your e-mail address
Subject: (leave blank)
Message: subscribe menieres_talk
Meniere's Coping List Group
To: coping@menieres.org
From: your e-mail address
Subject: subscribe
Message: (leave blank, no signature)

Fill in the blanks as instructed and send the e-mail. The mailing list computer will send back a message to announce that you are subscribed and to tell you how the group works and how to quit the list (unsubscribe). Keep these instructions; save them on disk, and print a copy. You will need these instructions later if you want to unsubscribe.

Don't write anything to a group that you would not want on the front page of your local newspaper. Most e-mails sent to an entire group or mailing list are saved for anyone to read at any time.

Summary

When you need more information about some aspect of Meniere's disease or its treatment, always begin with your physician. Other information about Meniere's can come from many sources representing many points of view.

Chapter 40

Success Stories

Many people can tell success stories about dealing with Meniere's disease. The following are especially good; they tell of people whose vertigo attacks stopped completely.

From Canada

"My story begins in 1985, the year I gave birth to my daughter. One day, totally out of the blue, I experienced two attacks of vertigo followed by one more the next day. Over the next four or five years there were no more vertigo episodes, but I did have tinnitus and a hearing loss in my left ear along with an occasional feeling of ear fullness.

"In 1990, the vertigo returned with a vengeance, absolutely turning my life upside down. The attacks were violent and frequent, making it impossible for me to function normally. After testing, my doctor told me I had Meniere's disease. Over the next few months we tried many medications (Stemetil, Serc, Gravol, Surmontil), all to no avail. As a matter of fact, the number of attacks increased during this time, and I could no longer work. The only success I had in my life was getting disability.

"My doctor told me shunt surgery might fix things, so during February of 1991 I had it done. Unfortunately it did not work for me, and I spent the next four years looking for relief. In 1992, I had streptomycin surgically placed into one of my ears, but the attacks continued. The next year brought allergy testing and the start of more than two years on the steroid prednisone. The prednisone helped somewhat but not enough, and I was experiencing serious weight gain and other problems steroids often cause. In the spring of 1995, I saw yet another otologist, who recommended and then did transtympanic gentamicin treatment.

"It is now the summer of 1997, and I have been free of vertigo since the summer of 1995. My ear is nearly deaf, and the tinnitus continues, but I am once again working and able to enjoy life. Of course I wish this success could have come sooner, but I'm happy to have it now. It does not get any better than being able to take your daughter to Disneyland and go on the rides together."

— P.P., telephone interview with the author, 1997

From Indiana

The first part of the story of Shereen D. Farber, Ph.D., OTR, was originally published in the May 1989 issue of the *American Journal of Occupational Therapy*. It appears here with permission.

"On Sept. 15, 1987, at 6 a.m., I jumped out of bed in my usual first light haste and promptly experienced unpleasant sensations. The room was whirling around me, making bipedal posture and locomotion a challenge. As I staggered across the room, enveloped by nausea, diaphoresis, and tachycardia, I prayed that I was in the middle of a bad dream and not really awake. My left ear felt full and painful, and within moments, I noted that certain head movements produced vertigo.

"I began the difficult task of learning new movement patterns that would enable me to accomplish necessary daily living tasks without landing on the floor. For example, after the vertigo started, the simple task of bending over to find my shoes on the floor would produce severe nausea with incapacitating dizziness. To compensate, I had to slowly lower myself to the floor, find my shoes, and then put them on while sitting. Getting into my slacks was difficult because I was used to balancing on one foot while inserting my other leg into the slacks. It presents a real challenge to balance on one leg when you cannot balance on two. As part of my initial movement strategies, I adopted a slow rate and rhythm for every activity. Since my normal movement patterns are brisk, I had to consciously slow my ventures. I quickly learned that if I turned my head, neck, and body to the left as a unit, the symptoms were reduced. I felt like the tin man in The Wizard of Oz. Daily living skills that I could no longer do in bipedal postures had to be done in a sitting or supine position.

"My otolaryngologist ordered a standard battery of vestibular and audiometric tests. Since I experienced symptoms only for a short time, none of my tests produced definitive findings. My doctor therefore outlined a conservative treatment regiment that began with dietary salt restriction.

"By the end of the first six-week period of salt restriction, I was markedly improved. It then became necessary to unlearn the compensation techniques I was using and relearn my normal motor patterns.

"At this point, I have no symptoms, but I continue to restrict my salt intake."

In a telephone interview in 1997, Dr. Farber said that in the years since her story first appeared in print she had not required surgery or other invasive treatments for her Meniere's disease. She attributed her success at keeping her symptoms under control to maintaining a diet low in sodium and fat and high in fresh vegetables, to avoiding great fatigue, and to craniosacral therapy.

From Colorado

"It started in late summer of 1973. I was finishing a project in Montreal and was getting ready to leave to go back to Denver. While packing, I dropped something, bent to pick it up, and suddenly became dizzy and nauseous to the point that I had to go back to bed for many hours. The next morning everything was fine, so I rescheduled my flight and came home. I believed I had nothing more than a stomach virus.

"I had no further problems for several months, then came an attack followed by others progressively more violent. Finally I visited a doctor, who after checking me over carefully and thoroughly said I might have Meniere's.

"He sent me to a specialist (an ear, nose, and throat doctor) who ran every conceivable test known at the time and concluded that I indeed had Meniere's.

"I continued to have attacks. One even caused me to fall over backwards, crush two vertebra, and become two inches shorter instantly. I got to the point where I was afraid to drive and had to rely on my good wife to take me everywhere. But I was able to continue to work.

"In 1984, I had to get a final physical before I could retire. During this exam, my doctor advised me to see a specialist who had just opened an office in the same medical complex. I did so. After about six months of testing, he advised that I was a good candidate for an operation whereby they would place a small pressure-relief valve in the inner ear so that the membrane would not rupture.

"The operation was done in late October 1984 and was a success even though I lost the hearing in the ear. I have not had any more Meniere's attacks since the operation. Unless one has gone through this, one cannot imagine the relief and gratefulness."

— G.L., letter to the author, 1997

Glossary

The following glossary briefly defines some of the terms used in this book. These and many other terms can best be understood in the context of the chapters in which they appear or by reviewing anatomical illustrations. For example, for definitions of surgical terms, see Chapter 29, "Surgery," and for definitions of professional specialties, see Chapter 37, "Who's Who in Otologic Health Care." To find the exact places in this book where certain terms are used, please refer to the Index.

Aftermath. Time immediately after an attack of Meniere's disease.

Air conduction. One of the two ways sound travels into the inner ear. The other way is bone conduction. By air conduction, sound strikes the tympanic membrane, and the resulting vibration travels to the inner ear via the middle ear bones and the oval window.

Ampulla. The bulbous end of a semicircular canal.

Antihistamine. A drug used to relieve the symptoms of allergies.

Ataxia. Lack of coordination.

Attack. The onset, usually dramatic, of an illness or symptoms. In this book, "attack" refers to a specific, intensely symptomatic time in the Meniere's cycle.

Audiogram. The "standard" hearing test that usually includes pure tones and speech.

Auditory. Refers to the sense of hearing.

Aural. Pertaining to the ear.

Auricle. The outside flap of the ear. Also called the pinna.

Autoimmune disease. Disease created when the body identifies some part of itself as foreign and attacks or rejects that part.

Balance. A state of repose between two or more antagonistic forces that exactly counteract each other.

Basilar membrane. Thin cochlear membrane upon which the organ of Corti rests.

Bone conduction. One of the two ways sound travels into the inner ear. The other is air conduction. Via bone conduction, sound strikes the skull, and the resulting vibration enters the cochlea directly or causes the middle ear bones to vibrate and to transmit the vibration into the inner ear via the oval window.

Brain stem. The part of the brain that performs motor, sensory, and reflex functions.

Burnout. See **Late-stage Meniere's disease.**

Caloric test. A test that requires irrigation of the ear canal with warm and/or cool water or air to measure vestibular functions.

Center of gravity. That point in a thing around which its weight is evenly distributed or balanced. Point of equilibrium.

Central nervous system. The brain and spinal cord.

Cerebellum. The part of the brain responsible for coordination.

Cerumen. Ear wax.

Cilia. Hairlike projections on the surfaces of some cells.

Cochlea. The end organ of hearing.

Computerized tomography (CT or CAT) scan. A scan using computers and X-rays to obtain highly detailed, three-dimensional information about body tissues and bone.

Conductive hearing loss. Hearing loss caused by problems with the transmission of sound from the outside world to the inner ear. This kind of hearing loss differs from sensorineural hearing loss, which usually arises from a problem inside the cochlea or in the auditory nerve.

Cupula. Gelatinous mass covering the hair cells in the ampulla of a semicircular canal.

Dandy's syndrome. A phrase sometimes used instead of *oscillopsia* to refer to the bouncing vision caused by bilateral vestibular loss.

Degeneration. Deterioration or impairment.

Disequilibrium. Vague sense of unsteadiness, imbalance, tilting, or bumping into things that can occur in association with vestibular problems.

Drop attack. *See* **Tumarkin's otolithic crisis.**

Dysautonomia. Dysfunction of the autonomic nervous system that can, on occasion, cause vertigo.

Ear drum. Common name for tympanic membrane. It forms the boundary between the outer and middle ears.

Electrolyte. Any chemical compound that, in solution, conducts electricity and is ionized by it. For example, sodium chloride (NaCl) ionizes in solution to become Na+ and Cl-.

Electronystagmography (ENG). A method of measuring eye movements. A battery of ENG tests, including the caloric ENG, may be used to assess relationships between the eyes and the vestibular system and help diagnose the cause of dizziness or vertigo.

Endolymph. Fluid within the membranous labyrinth of the inner ear.

Endolymphatic hydrops. Excessive amount of endolymph. Increased pressure from this endolymph can damage any part of the vestibular apparatus or the cochlea.

Equilibrium. State of repose between two or more antagonistic forces that exactly counteract each other.

Eustachian tube. Hourglass-shaped tube connecting the middle ear with the area of the throat behind the nose.

Fistula. Abnormal opening from one internal organ to another or leading to a surface. Fistulas can occur between the inner ear and the middle ear.

Gait. Manner of walking.

Giddiness. Dizziness; lightheadedness.

Hallpike test. A test to see if nystagmus occurs during certain changes in head position. It is useful in diagnosing BPPV.

Hyperacusis. Abnormal sensitivity to sound. It does not usually include vertigo caused by sound.

Idiopathic. Of unknown cause.

Incus. One of three middle ear bones. Also called the anvil, it lies between the malleus and the stapes.

Inner ear. Fluid-filled system of chambers and passageways encased in the temporal bone. The inner ear includes the end organs of hearing and balance and is also called the labyrinth.

Ion. Atom or group of atoms carrying an electric charge.

Labyrinth. Complex series of chambers and passageways of the inner ear, including the hearing and balance parts.

Labyrinthitis. Inflammation of the labyrinth or part of it.

Late-stage Meniere's disease. Time in the course of Meniere's disease when the violent episodes of vertigo stop and are replaced by a sometimes constant unsteadiness or imbalance. Sometimes referred to as burnout.

Macula. In the inner ear, a tiny area of neural tissue in the saccule or utricle.

Magnetic resonance imaging (MRI). Diagnostic tool that produces cross-sectional images of parts of the body. An MRI of the brain can reveal the presence of tumors, stroke damage, and some other abnormalities.

Malleus. Outermost of the three ossicles (middle-ear bones). It is sometimes called the hammer.

Mastoid. Bone, partly filled with air spaces, located behind the ear.

Meniere's cycle. Recurring pattern of variable symptoms—warning, attack, aftermath, and remission—that characterizes Meniere's disease.

Meniere's disease. Idiopathic syndrome of endolymphatic hydrops.

Middle ear. Part of the ear that reaches from the ear drum to the outer surfaces of the oval and round windows.

Modiolus. A cone-shaped core of spongy bone that the cochlea is wrapped around.

Motion intolerance. Strong symptoms such as vertigo or nausea arising from head movement. These symptoms may cause avoidance of movement.

Neurotransmitter. Chemical that carries a nerve signal.

Nystagmus. Abnormal eye jerking.

Organ of Corti. Hearing end organ.

Oscillopsia. Visual illusion that stationary objects are bobbing to and fro, back and forth, or up and down.

Ossicles. The three tiny bones of the middle ear.

Otic capsule. Outer shell of the bony labyrinth.

Otitis media. Inflammation of the middle ear.

Otoliths. Calcium carbonate crystals stuck to the otolithic membrane of the utricle and saccule. Sometimes also called *ear rocks*.

Otolithic membrane. Gelatinous-like material resting on the hair cells of the utricle or saccule.

Oval window. One of two covered openings between the middle ear and the inner ear.

Perilymph. Fluid surrounding and cushioning the membranous labyrinth.

Pinna. External, visible part of the ear. Also called the *auricle*.

Proprioception. Gathering information via sensors in muscles, tendons, joints, ligaments, and connective tissue. The information is about gravity, body position, external surfaces, and the length and motion of the muscles and joints.

Reissner's membrane. The upper membrane of the scala media of the cochlea.

Remission. Time of reduced or absent symptoms between Meniere's attacks.

Round window. Membrane-covered opening between the inner ear and the middle ear.

Saccule. Inner ear chamber containing hair cells.

Scala media. The cochlear duct, including the organ of Corti.

Scala tympani. One of three channels running the length of the cochlea.

Scala vestibuli. One of three channels running the length of the cochlea.

Semicircular canal. Curved inner ear structure containing an organ that detects angular head movement.

Sensorineural hearing loss. Hearing loss caused by damage to the cochlea or the vestibulo-cochlear nerve. This used to be referred to simply as "nerve loss." This kind of hearing loss differs from conductive hearing loss, which arises from a problem with the transmission of sound from the outside world to the inner ear.

Sixth sense. The sense of balance.

Spatial disorientation. Confusion about one's position in space. This might include confusion about the location of vertical and horizontal

Syncope. Fainting or passing out.

Spinal tap. Removal of fluid from the spinal column in order to reveal information about the spinal cord and brain. Also called *lumbar puncture.*

Stapes. The innermost of the three middle-ear bones. It is sometimes referred to as the *stirrup* because of its shape.

Stria vascularis. One of the walls of the scala media of the cochlea.

Syndrome: All of the signs and symptoms of a disease process taken together and constituting the picture of the disease.

Tectorial membrane. Gelatinous mass located immediately above the hair cells in the organ of Corti.

Temporal bone. The part of the skull in which the inner ear is located.

Tinnitus. Hissing, ringing, or other abnormal noises in the ears. Commonly called "ringing in the ears."

Traveling wave. Wave of movement caused by a sound wave entering the inner ear.

Tullio phenomenon. Vertigo and/or nystagmus caused by a loud sound.

Tumarkin's otolithic crisis. Falling on the ground or floor without any warning because of sudden loss of balance. *See also* **Drop attack.**

Tympanic membrane. Ear drum.

Utricle. Inner ear chamber containing hair cells.

Vertigo. Perception of movement (either of yourself or of objects around you) that is not occurring or is occurring differently from what you perceive.

Vestibular. Related to the balance parts of the inner ear and related structures.

Vestibular ocular reflex (VOR). Involuntary eye movements caused by stimulating the vestibular system.

Vestibulo-cochlear nerve. Nerve from the brain that is essential to the senses of hearing and balance. Also called *eighth cranial nerve, auditory nerve, or acoustic nerve.*

Warning. Time immediately before an attack of Meniere's disease during which telltale symptoms are experienced.

Index

Bold page numbers refer to definitions; italic page numbers refer to illustrations.

B

T